Compassion

Compassion
The essence of palliative and end-of-life care

Philip J Larkin

Professor of Clinical Nursing (Palliative Care),
UCD School of Nursing,
Midwifery and Health Systems and
Our Lady's Hospice and Care Services,
Harold's Cross, Dublin

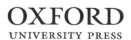
OXFORD
UNIVERSITY PRESS

OXFORD
UNIVERSITY PRESS

Great Clarendon Street, Oxford, OX2 6DP,
United Kingdom

Oxford University Press is a department of the University of Oxford.
It furthers the University's objective of excellence in research, scholarship,
and education by publishing worldwide. Oxford is a registered trade mark of
Oxford University Press in the UK and in certain other countries

© Oxford University Press 2016

The moral rights of the author have been asserted

First Edition published in 2016

Impression: 1

Published in the United States of America by Oxford University Press
198 Madison Avenue, New York, NY 10016, United States of America

British Library Cataloguing in Publication Data

Data available

Library of Congress Control Number: 2015941537

ISBN 978–0–19–870331–0

Printed in Great Britain by
Clays Ltd, St Ives plc

This book is dedicated to patients and families whose living with dying experience calls for a truly compassionate response and to those who respond to that call through loving wisdom and 'care-full' practice.

Foreword

Compassion is a powerful therapeutic tool. When used wisely, with sincerity, and in the context of evidenced-based practice, it is exactly what all health and social care workers should aspire to provide. Compassion creates an environment of safety, where trust can be built in an interpersonal relationship between patients, their families, and health care professionals. This is crucial for sustaining hope in times of crisis and threat, especially in palliative care where the consciousness of imminent loss is ever-present. The sense that a patient is truly the focus of attention, rather than their disease process, medication regime, or blood test results, is the essence of person-centred care. Perhaps even more important is the way compassion can enhance relationships. For example, just 'being heard' as a person (not a patient, a disease, or a set of complex symptoms) may be transformative. Patient and family accounts demonstrate that the simple fact of being acknowledged as a person with a name and remembered as an individual with a life story outside the confines of their disease is life-enhancing. This attention to personhood (in both patient and family member) is especially salient during end-of-life care when health professionals' communication and care practices become memorized by those who witness the dying.

This book is focused on exploring aspects of the lived experience of compassion through the narrative accounts of some of the most inspirational clinicians working in palliative care globally. It is wonderful that Professor Philip J Larkin has captured the power of story using biographical narratives to undertake this important analysis of compassion. Like Dame Cicely Saunders, who used a number of evocative stories to illustrate the philosophy of her new vision for terminal care, Professor Larkin has used the genre of narrative to construct his book. Therefore the book can be read in a number of different ways: as a simple account of the interesting lives of some key leaders in the palliative care field, as a way to engage with reflective practice, or as an insightful academic analysis of the concept of compassion. There is virtue in and something to be gained from each way of reading the text, so multiple readings may be rewarded.

Compassion is a continuous process of engagement and meaning making, occurring both consciously and unconsciously, in clinical practice. In contrast, are there some environments or contexts where it is extremely difficult to enact compassion? It is all too easy to blame the individual nurse or doctor as lacking in compassion when structural or organizational factors conspire to place excessive demands upon them: for example, very high workloads, too many demands, little emotional support, leadership focused upon completion of tasks or cost-saving goals, lack of training in communication skills, little effective modelling and valuing of psychosocial care as an intrinsic component of all good health care. How then can individuals foster and sustain the compassion that most brought with them as novice practitioners?

This book offers some wonderful examples of how compassion can be demonstrated and taught. Compassion is central to medical, nursing, and other types of health and social care, especially in the setting of progressive disease that will end in the patient's death and reside in the memory of family and friends. This is a necessary book; its messages hopefully will stay long in your memory, too.

Professor Sheila Payne
Co-Director, International Observatory on End-of-Life Care
Lancaster University, United Kingdom
President, European Association for Palliative Care

Preface

Two things led to the decision to write this book. First, compassion appears to be an important expectation in the delivery of health care, but the evidence for that in practice is nebulous. As a word, it peppers health care literature in terms of the expectations and outcomes of the practice of health care professionals. As a nurse, I was very aware that the ideal of compassion is deeply embedded in nursing philosophy but rarely discussed or debated. As an educator, the study of compassion does not easily offer the defined measurable learning outcomes expected from robust curricula. I was also keen to explore if the mission statements of many clinics, hospitals, and hospices using the term *compassion* to express their aspirations for care delivery translated from the plaque on the wall to the practice at the bedside.

For palliative and end-of-life care, it would almost be sacrilegious to suggest that such care without compassion is even possible. Yet after 25 years as a practitioner in the field, I would find it difficult to pinpoint what makes a palliative care practitioner compassionate, how that is known or demonstrated, or even why that should be.

Overall, it seems that compassion is something valuable and warranted and yet somewhat intangible.

The second reason that prompted this book was a growing concern within the health care literature and the media that compassion has been lost in the care of dying people. The recent review of the Liverpool Care Pathway for Dying Patients (to give its full title), the subsequent findings of professional misconduct and poor clinical practice in the Mid Staffordshire NHS Foundation Trust Public Inquiry (the Francis Report), as well as UK media and health literature reports of uncaring and indifferent practice by health care professionals have put the care offered in a palliative and end-of-life context to the test, with particular criticism levelled against the nursing profession. Lessons from the UK experience suggest reflection on the concept of compassion may serve that current debate.

A tangential argument to this is that compassion has in some way been eroded or marginalized in the practice of caring for people who are dying because of an over-reliance on clinical and technological intervention, contrary to the ideal of quality and not quantity of life. This may have been a particular challenge for those who, like me, crossed over from the hospice model to palliative care as an intervention which can be offered along the disease trajectory and not simply a best-practice model for end-of-life care. During the writing of this book, I was fortunate to be awarded a Fulbright Scholarship which enabled me to spend five months with the palliative care service in the renowned Dana-Farber Cancer Institute (DFCI) in Boston. This time exposed me to the work of a team providing palliative care in an environment that clearly has cure as its raison-d'être (but compassion in its strapline!). I attended meetings, grand rounds, conferences, and presentations; observed clinicians in practice; saw how clinical decisions were made; attended family meetings; and engaged in interviews and dialogue with a range of clinicians and practitioners about the meaning of providing compassionate palliative care. I also had the privilege of attending Schwartz Center rounds (http://www.theschwartzcenter.org) which focus on compassionate health care. Particularly poignant were those held in memory of the Boston Marathon bombings, whose first anniversary took place while I was living in Boston. Above all, I wrote and documented what I experienced.

The team that I met worked from a spirit of clinical excellence, wise judgement, and tenacity in approach to ensure all patients and their families received excellence in care. As I was exposed to different models of practice and caregiving at DFCI, it became apparent that compassionate palliative care is about negotiating a fundamental shift in the priorities and goals across the experience of living towards the possibility of death, managed through relationship, respect for the centrality of the patient and family in decision-making, and, of course, compassion. As an example of how professional palliative care can be modelled, DFCI offers both vision and leadership. I am forever grateful for what I learnt from them about the practice of compassionate palliative care.

A further observation which sparked my enthusiasm for this book was the rise of palliative care literature in relation to compassionate practice and teaching from a Buddhist perspective, evident in the range of peer-reviewed journal articles, books, and grey literature, in which I include popular self-help literature. Of all the major faiths in the world, Buddhism shares the most visible exploration of compassion as a way to address suffering at end of life in meaningful and practical ways.

However, as contributors to this book attest, the founding of the modern hospice movement by Cicely Saunders in the 1960s was based on a strong Christian perspective clearly as seen in the early letters published in the edited book by David Clark in 2005. Her publication from 2003, *Watch with Me*, had a clear influence on a number of the contributors to this book. There seems to be some concern that the foundation of this early vision and direction has been 'airbrushed' out of the history and is worthy of at least a distinguished mention.

This is not to say that a variety of world philosophical and theological perspectives are not meaningful, just that a thoughtful discourse on compassion in palliative care should not obscure the roots in search of the bloom.

This book is based on a series of interviews conducted between 2013 and 2014 with a range of international expert clinicians who live the practice of compassionate palliative and end-of-life care on a daily basis. The people in this book are the opinion leaders, founders, and pioneers who have carried the mission of Cicely Saunders across the world, from a range of disciplines and practice perspectives. Interviews were either face-to-face or by telephone. Many sent additional resources, documents, thoughts, and ideas as the writing progressed. All generated a wealth of textual data which was reformulated into the various chapters.

Following a brief personal introduction which asks what compassion means, each of the subsequent chapters presents the reflections of the contributor on the topic of compassionate care. Respecting the Christian tradition of Cicely Saunders, a description of compassion by the author and Roman Catholic priest Henri Nouwen (see chapter 1) was offered as a catalyst for conversation on the practice of palliative and end-of-life care. Each chapter concludes with a commentary which draws together key themes raised in the context of wider literature, reflections for practice, as well as references and web resources. For this reason, and the accessibility of its e-book format, I hope the content will be of interest to students, practitioners, and educators alike. In terms of reference materials used for this book, two stand out for special mention. The e-book *Compassion: Bridging Practice and Science* (2013) is edited by Tania Singer and Matthias Bolz from the Max Planck Institute in Leipzig. Arising from a symposium in Berlin, this book represents the collective wisdom of neuroscientists, artists, clinicians, psychologists, and contemplatives (such as Buddhist monks and Zen masters) on how to instil compassion in society at large. As such, it is one of the most comprehensive and contemporary resources for the study of compassion. The book is available as a free download (http://www.compassion-training.org) and is compelling reading.

The second resource was the collected works of theologian and author Karen Armstrong and, in particular, the Charter for Compassion (http://charterfor-compassion.org) which calls on religious and secular traditions to embrace a shared dialogue of equality and interdependence. Both are valuable resources within which to understand the messages of this book.

As you begin this book, I am mindful of a phrase in the Irish language recently cited by the president of Ireland, Dr Michael D. Higgins, during an historic first state visit to England from the Republic of Ireland. The translation of the phrase, 'to live in the shadow and shelter of each other' (*ar scáth a chéile a mhairimíd*), reflects a complex history and relationship between two countries which exist side-by-side. It also speaks to the interconnectedness of people by virtue of a shared humanity and that alone speaks to the importance of compassion in society and in the care we give to those for whom the expectation of life is limited and for which we, as palliative care practitioners, hold responsibility. As Henri Nouwen contends, 'You are the difference you make' (Nouwen et al. 1982: 19).

Philip J Larkin

Acknowledgements

This book is a collaborative effort and a number of people warrant mention and thanks for helping to bring it to fruition.

I wish to thank all those who gave of their time, expertise, and wisdom to contribute to the various chapters in this book. Your willingness to take part, respond to, review, and revise scripts and guide on further resources and materials for reflection was much appreciated. This book is only here because of your contribution. I would like to acknowledge the support of the Dana-Farber Cancer Institute and, in particular, the director of the Psychosocial Oncology and Palliative Care Division, Dr Susan Block, for agreeing to sponsor my Fulbright scholarship in medical science and for offering study resources and space to conduct the academic work. Special thanks are due to Dr Janet Abrahm, attending physician in the Division of Adult Palliative Care, who guided me safely through the Dana-Farber experience and also contributed to the book. I am of course also grateful to the Fulbright Commission of Ireland who saw the potential for this work, sponsored my scholarship visit to Boston, and gave me the experience of what it means to be a Fulbrighter. My thanks also to Dr Martin McNamara, School of Nursing and Midwifery, University College Dublin, and Ms. Mo Flynn, latterly CEO, Our Lady's Hospice and Care Services, Harold's Cross, for giving me the opportunity to take up the scholarship. I would also like to thank Caroline Smith and Nicola Wilson at Oxford University Press for agreeing to take a chance on something new in their publishing style and for the help with bringing this to the final stages of completion.

I also want to express my sincere thanks to my personal assistant, Ms. Eleanor Blake at Our Lady's Hospice and Care Services, Harold's Cross, Dublin, for her incredible capacity to manage the process of appointments, time zones, skilful transcription, follow-up, and generally keeping me on track. I am certain that this book would not have happened without her guiding hand. I acknowledge also Ms. Debbie Emerson who also assisted with transcription services.

Throughout this book, names in case exemplars are either anonymized at the request of the contributor or published with permission of the person or family. Any factual errors or omissions in this book are mine alone.

Contents

Chapter 1

Philip J Larkin—Compassion: a conceptual reading for palliative and end-of-life care

Introduction to compassion

Compassion has roots in many academic disciplines: philosophy, theology, sociology, psychology, and virtue ethics. It can be complex to define and objectify in terms of an expected response or outcome to a given situation. Depending on the particular stance taken, compassion is an innate trait of humanity, a skill or attribute to be developed, or a way of being based on specific spiritual life perspectives. Within palliative and end-of-life care, the goal to address suffering and its impact on physical, psychosocial, and spiritual well-being resonates with the expression of compassion, a deeper understanding of which may help in exploring contemporary clinical practice. This brief introduction orientates the reader to the wider academic discourse on compassion and provides a context for the chapters which follow. By its nature, this introduction is a guide to key questions rather than a comprehensive debate on the topic (see also Larkin 2011: 154). There is also a considerable body of work which looks at the issues of burnout and compassion fatigue in palliative care. Although alluded to by some contributors, these issues are not addressed to any significant extent in this volume.

The language of compassion

Providing a global definition of compassion is complex because of its own intrinsic moral and spiritual values (Schantz 2007). There is something inherently personal about compassion which speaks to our own world views and life history. Sasser and Puchalski (2010) consider that compassion 'provides the unspoken language to address unspeakable suffering' (p. 937). As such, it also speaks to founding ideals of hospice and palliative care, both historically and contemporaneously (Davidson 2014; Clark 2005).

From their evolutionary analysis, Goetz et al. (2010) consider compassion as an affective experience with the purpose to 'facilitate co-operation and care for the weak' (p. 351). Its etymological definition as 'suffering together with an-other', derived from *com* (together with) and *pati* (to suffer) (http://www.oed.com), resonates with palliative care as a practice which works to address the tripartite 'total pain' approach, where attentiveness to physical pain enables the less tangible psychological, social, and spiritual suffering to be broached. Key to this is relationship, a deep respect for human nature and a desire to do every-thing possible to relieve that suffering (Bergum 2004; Pask 2003). Personhood of the patient and family as they live their life in the context of life-limiting ill-ness is a paramount consideration, particularly in light of the growing discourse around healing and holistic models of practice for living life in connection (Bre-itbart 2008; Randall & Downie 2006; Wishart 2005; Mount & Kearney 2003).

Compassion presupposes three main elements (Nussbaum 2001). The suffer-ing must be significant. It should be largely unmerited. Most important, it could be potentially experienced by the one observing the suffering. Hence, intercon-nectedness leads to reaching out of one to the other in a desire to care. As Gal-lagher (2009) phrased it, 'Compassion responds to the pain it can see with its eyes, and its natural expression is the embrace of care' (p. 239).

Innovative neuroscience using diagnostic imaging now suggests that there is evidence of a significant neurological connection between persons when suffer-ing is perceived (Singer & Bolz 2013). This favours Nussbaum's (1996) fourth constituent to compassion, *eudaimonia* or 'flourishing happiness'. We are well when happy, successful, and content, and so we desire this for ourselves and others. There are nuances to be considered in the compassion discourse. For example, is compassion qualitatively different if experienced remotely (a natu-ral disaster in another country shown on television) or as the result of self-in-flicted injury (lung cancer due to smoking) (Gallagher 2009)? Even the proposition that compassion is innate is challenged since choice is involved; it may be oriented towards the community rather than towards an individual (Kellehear 2013; Schantz 2007; Gyatso 2002). Such are the 'compassionate co-nundrums' posited by Gallagher (2013).

Compassion mirrors complex concepts in their own right, including empa-thy, sympathy, and pity. Compassion has been addressed in the context of power (Wishart 2005), silence (Back et al. 2009), love (Leathard 2004), presence (Sabo 2011), care (Dewar et al. 2014), altruism (Saslow et al. 2013), and as po-litical virtue (Whitebrook 2002).

Empathy has been the subject of significant study, particularly from the perspec-tive of social neuroscience, philosophy, and medicine (Svaenus 2014; Agosta 2014; Bornemark 2014; Neff & Germer 2013; Reiss et al. 2012). Empathy enables the cli-nician to see suffering more clearly and assists in the ethical decision-making pro-cess (Svaenus 2014). However, empathy alone is insufficient for real compassion to exist and may distance rather than deepen a compassionate connection (Dalai Lama 2005; Hayward 2005). Patterns of sympathy and pity have also seen critique in the literature, the former for its overtly subjective nature which fails to respond coherently to the needs of the other and the latter for failing to act decisively to assist the sufferer to seek solutions to their plight (Gallagher 2009; Crisp 2008; Barad 2007; Frazer 2006; Keaty 2005). It is therefore evident that multiple perspectives shape our understanding of compassion and offer a variety of ways to consider its application to palliative and end-of-life care.

Compassion in global wisdom traditions

Compassion is deeply rooted in faith and wisdom traditions across the world. Archetypal images such as the Christian *Good Samaritan* painted by George Frederick Watts (see Figure 1.1) or the Buddhist bodhisattva of compassion *Avalokitesvara* ('Lord who looks down'), known in China as *Guānyīn* (goddess of mercy), both speak to the importance of compassion as a visible representation of a response to suffering. Watts's work, which shows a wounded man leaning on the Samaritan for support and aid in his ordeal, is derived from strong Christian values. These values underpin many of his works and are perhaps reminiscent of a similar ethos of Christian value in the vision of Cicely Saunders for hospice care.

The author and theologian Karen Armstrong, who has addressed the importance of compassion as a way to build a more tolerant society (Armstrong 2011, see also http://www.charterforcompassion.org), cites the Golden Rule (Confucius 551–479 BCE) as the abiding principle which links to the compassionate core of all faith-based traditions (Muhammad 2014; Owain Hughes 2013; Delio 2005; Griffiths 2001; Sears 1998; Hanh 1995). Buddhist perspectives on compassion seem to have gained particular visibility in the body of literature related to the field of death, dying, and palliative and end-of-life care (Singer & Bolz 2013; Masel et al. 2012; Rinpoche et al. 2012; Halifax, 2011; Ikeda 2004). The deeply valuable roots of Cicely Saunders's (2003) strong Christian belief as a catalyst for her work equally merits attention, a point raised by many contributors.

In the *Summa Theologica*, Thomas Aquinas (1225–1274) treats compassion and mercy as synonymous; charity (*caritas*) is a theological virtue and mercy as responding to another's unhappiness (*misericordia*). Similar perspectives on Christian love, stewardship, human dignity, the sanctity of life, justice, and finitude also link to messages of compassion and palliative and end-of-life care (Leathard 2004; Dodds 1991; Sevensky 1983). Arguably, love and compassion are essential for the survival of humanity (Halifax 2011). The description of compassion taken from Nouwen et al (1982), provided opportunity to consider if this

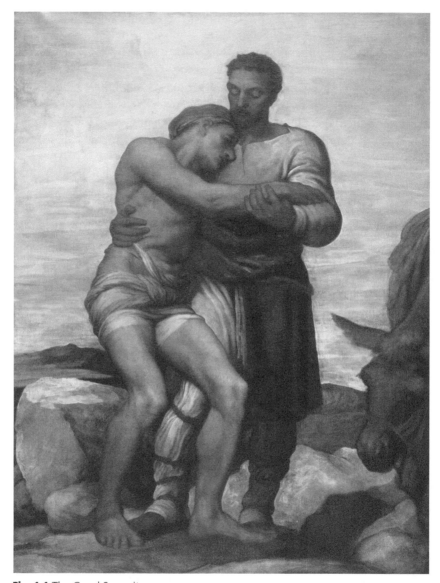

Fig. 1.1 The Good Samaritan.

The Good Samaritan, 1852 (oil on canvas), Watts, George Frederick (1817–1904) /Manchester Art Gallery, UK/The Bridgeman Art Library.

resonated with contributors' understanding and experience of compassion: 'Compassion asks us to go where it hurts, to enter into places of pain, to share in brokenness, fear, confusion and anguish. . . . Compassion means full immersion in the condition of being human' (Nouwen et al. 1982: 4).

Here, true compassion is experienced physically (*Splangchnizomai*, 'within the gut'), leading to action that responds to another's suffering. Compassion as a guide to our inner conscience can govern clinical discernment on when or how to act or not act in certain circumstances, respecting that death may be the inevitable outcome of human existence which cannot be avoided. How this definition speaks as a guiding principle for practice opens a wider debate on the meaning of pain, the challenge of facing suffering, and what it means to be human in the context of clinical care delivery.

Compassion perspectives on palliative and end-of-life care

Whether there is a specific relationship between compassion and palliative and end-of-life care and, if so, what is that relationship and how is it expressed, is debatable. The suggestion that compassion is the essence of palliative and end-of-life care is equally contentious. It could be taken to mean, ipso facto, that it cannot apply to any other type of care. This is clearly not the case.

The World Health Organisation's (2002) revised definition of palliative care (http://www.who.int/cancer/palliative/definition/en) seems to mark a transition point from the historical hospice-based, cancer-orientated approach to the more integrative approach, applicable across a wide range of chronic and life-limiting illness, which it has now become. This redefinition is not without criticism (Randall & Downie 2006). In seeking a new language to describe what palliative care is *not* (i.e. a terminal care service only for the last days and weeks of life), it is suggested that the relationship between palliative care and dying is no longer clear (Illhardt 2001). Given that palliative care is both a philosophy of caring and a model of service delivery, the extent to which it remains rooted in the founding ideals of compassionate care warrant review. There are a number of false assumptions in the way in which this transition has been interpreted, one of which is that Cicely Saunders's vision was antithetical to the idea of integrated care. Rather, as evidenced in her own writings (Clark 2005), she sought to implant an idea of caring in a different way, not simply related to a building. The need for the care of dying people in both hospital and community was always envisioned as a response to need as the philosophy and practice developed. Therefore, the idea that this approach to care was ultimately transferable across systems was not contradictory. Saunders's vision for hospice care took place at a time of profound change within the British health care system and the advent of the National Health Service which had its critics, both then and now (Mandlestam 2006; Pollock 2004; Rivett 1998). The model that she perceived of best care at end of life—largely shaped by her exposure to care in the voluntary sector—was appealing in a time of organizational turmoil. It provided an ethos that offered a bounded structure for people coming to terms with the fact that 'through acceptance of the life one has lived comes acceptance of death' (Breitbart 2008: 212).

Integration into mainstream health care has shaped the development of palliative care services across many countries, including those that also espouse the hospice model, and has been, by and large, successful. However, delivering compassionate palliative care presents challenges in health systems that are essentially fiscally motivated, insurance-driven, and consumerist. The work of Robin Youngson in the Compassion in Health care movement (see https:// www.heartsinhealthcare.org) attests to this. At the time of writing this chapter while based in the Dana-Farber Cancer Institute in Boston, the changing face of US health care with the introduction of the Affordable Care Act (http:// www.hhs.gov/healthcare/rights) offered a further perspective to explore the complexity of compassionate care delivery. The UK experience is salutatory. Key reports such as the Mid-Staffordshire NHS Foundation Trust Public Inquiry (the Francis Report; http://www.midstaffspublicinquiry.com) and the review of the Liverpool Care Pathway for Dying Patients (https://www.gov.uk/ government/publications/review-of-liverpool-care-pathway-for-dying-patents) have delivered compelling messages about poor practice and inadequate clinical standards directly relevant to the place of compassion in palliative and end-of-life care. Media reports and the wider health care literature all use compassion as an indicator by which poor clinical standards, neglect, and lack of care has been judged (Newdick & Danbury 2013; Gallagher 2013; Paley 2013). Nursing as a profession seems to have been a particular target, with calls that compassion should be a professional requirement within the UK code of conduct and that compassion should be a key criterion for recruitment (Smajdor 2013; Duffin 2013; Bradshaw 2009). Therefore, compassion does seem to have some essential quality that we seek, particularly when directed towards care groups such as the vulnerable elderly and those facing end of life.

Compelled to action—some final thoughts on compassion

Nouwen's argument contends that feeling compassion is not enough. The Good Samaritan is compelled to intervene and take action. Cicely Saunders's belief that 'the way care is given can reach the most hidden places' (Saunders 1996) championed palliative care as making a difference to lives by a willingness to engage carefully and purposefully to meet needs, both visible and obscured. When the humanity and vulnerability of the practitioner and the patient are held in equal measure, a core message for both compassion and palliative and end-of-life care is confirmed—'You are the difference you make' (Nouwen et al. 1982). Compassion requires resilience, fortitude, and sometimes risk-taking, but always tenacity and determination. In the opening stanza of 'Cry Out in Your Weakness' (Mathnawi II), the thirteenth-century Sufi poet and mystic Jallāl ad-Dīn Rumi writes:

> A dragon was pulling a bear into its terrible mouth
> A courageous man went and rescued the bear.
> There are such helpers in the world, who rush to save
> anyone who cries out. Like mercy itself,
> they run toward the screaming.
> And they can't be bought off.
> If you were to ask one of those, 'Why did you come
> so quickly?' he or she would say, 'Because I heard your helplessness.'
> Rumi, the 13th Century mystic, reproduced from Banks C., *Delicious Laughter:*
> *Rambunctious teaching stories from the Mathnawi Jelaluddin Rumi*, Maypop, USA,
> Copyright © 1990. Translated by and reproduced with permission of Coleman Banks.

The energy of the helpers expressed here speaks to the action of compassion beyond any sense or feeling associated with it. Ram Dass and Mirabai Bush (1992) ask what is within us as human beings that responds to the needs of others. To answer that, the contributors to this book, all expert clinicians in palliative care, were asked to consider three questions: what it means to be a compassionate practitioner of palliative and end-of-life care, how that was demonstrated and interpreted in practice though case examples, and how compassion can be fostered and sustained for the next generation of practitioners. A descriptor of compassion as cited earlier in this chapter by Nouwen et al. 1982 (p. 4) was used to begin dialogue. The term *palliative and end-of-life care* was used to emphasize the continuation of care from early intervention through to the process of death. Each contributor described their reasons and motivations for coming into the clinical field. The place of a faith-based or spiritual practice for the expression of compassion in palliative and end-of-life care was discussed, as was each contributor's approach to the teaching of compassion. How important these messages are for palliative and end-of-life care practitioners is what this book is about. The practice wisdom of this book's contributors seeks to unpack that question in order to decide if compassion is indeed the essence of palliative and end-of-life care.

Further reading

Agosta L (2014) A rumor of empathy: reconstructing Heidegger's contribution to empathy and empathic clinical practice. Medicine, Health Care and Philosophy, 17(2): 281–292.

Armstrong K (2011) Twelve steps to a compassionate life. New York: Anchor.

Back AL, Bauer-Wu SM, Rushton C, Halifax J (2009) Compassionate silence in the patient-clinician encounter: a contemplative approach. Journal of Palliative Medicine, **12**(12), 1113–1117.

Barad J (2007) The understanding and experience of compassion: Aquinas and the Dalai Lama. Buddhist-Christian Studies, **27**, 11–29.

Bergum V (2003) Relational Pedagogy. Embodiment, Improvisation and Interdependence. Nursing Philosophy, **4**(2), 121–128.

Bergum V (2004) Relational ethics in nursing. In J Storch et al. (eds), Toward a moral horizon: nursing ethics for leadership and practice. Toronto, ON: Prentice Hall. 485–503.

Bornemark J (2014) The genesis of empathy in human development: A phenomenological reconstruction. Medicine, Health Care and Philosophy, **17**(2), 259–268.

Bradshaw A (2009) Measuring nursing care and compassion: The McDonaldised Nurse. Journal of Medical Ethics, **35**(8), 465–468.

Breitbart W (2008) Thoughts on the goals of psychosocial palliative care. Palliative and Supportive Care, **6**, 211–212.

Clark D (2005) Cicely Saunders: founder of the hospice movement. Selected letters 1959–1999. Oxford: Oxford University Press.

Crisp R (2008) Compassion and beyond. Ethical Theory, Morality and Practice, **11**, 233–246.

Dalai Lama (2005) How to expand love: widening the circle of loving relationships. New York: Atria.

Dass R, Bush M (1992) Compassion in action: setting out on the path of service. New York: Bell Tower.

Davidson G (2014) The hospice: development and administration. Oxford: Routledge.

Delio I (2005) Compassion: living in the spirit of St Francis. Cincinnati, OH: Franciscan Media

Dewar B, Adamson E, Smith S, Surfleet J, King L (2014) Clarifying misconceptions about compassionate care. Journal of Advanced Nursing, **70**(8), 1738–1747.

Dodds M (1991) Thomas Aquinas, human suffering and the unchanging God of love. Theological Studies, **52**, 330–344.

Duffin C (2013) Nurses could be struck off by NMC for failing to show compassion, Nursing Standard, **27**(46), 2–3.

Frazer ML (2006) The compassion of Zarathustra: Nietzsche on sympathy and strength. The review of politics, **68**(1), 49–78.

Gallagher A (2013) Compassion conundrums. Nursing Ethics, **20**(8), 849–850.

Gallagher P (2009) The grounding of forgiveness: Martha Nussbaum on compassion and mercy. American Journal of Economics and Sociology, **68**(1), 231–252.

Goetz JL, Keltner D, Simon-Thomas E (2010) Compassion: an evolutionary analysis and empirical review. Psychological Bulletin, **136**(3), 351–374.

Griffiths B (2001) River of compassion. Springfield, IL: Templegate.

Gyatso, GK (2002) Universal compassion: inspiring solutions for difficult times. New York: Tharpa.

Halifax J (2011) The precious necessity of compassion. Journal of Pain and Symptom Management, **41**(1), 146–152.

Hanh TN (1995) Living Buddha, living Christ. New York: Riverhead.

Hayward R (2005) Historical Keywords – Empathy. Lancet, **366**(9491), 1071.

Ikeda D (2004) Unlocking the mysteries of birth and death . . . and everything in between: a Buddhist view of life. Santa Monica, CA: Middleway Press.

Illhardt FJ (2001) Scope and demarcation of palliative care In H Ten Have, R Janssens (eds) Palliative care in Europe: concepts and policies. Amsterdam: IOS Press. 109–116.

Keaty A (2005) The Christian Virtue of Mercy: Aquinas' transformation of Aristotelian Pity. The Heythrop Journal, **46**(2), 181–198.

Kellehear A (2013) Compassionate communities: end-of-life care as everyone's responsibility. QJM, **106**, 1071–1075.

Larkin P (2011) Compassion: the essence of end-of-life care. In I Renzenbrink (ed) Caregiver stress and staff support in illness, dying and bereavement. Oxford: Oxford University Press.

Leathard HL (2004) The nature of being: a Thomistic perspective related to health and healing. Spirituality and Health International, **5**(2), 107–115.

Mandelstam M (2006) Betraying the NHS: health abandoned. London: Jessica Kingsley.

Masel EK, Schur S, Watzske HH (2012) Life is uncertain, death is certain: Buddhism and palliative care. Journal of Pain and Symptom Management, **44**(2), 307–312.

Mount B, Kearney M (2003) Healing and palliative care: charting our way forward. Palliative Medicine, **17**, 657–658.

Muhammad T (2014) Islam on mercy and compassion. London: Minhaj-Ul-Quran.

Neff K, Germer C (2013) Being kind to yourself: the science of self-compassion. In T Singer, M Bolz (eds) Compassion: bridging practice and science. Munich: Max Planck Society. 492–499.

Newdick C, Danbury C (2013) Culture, compassion and clinical neglect: Probity in the NHS after Mid Staffordshire. Journal of Medical Ethics, Published Online First, 08.04.14, doi.1010.1136/medethics.2012-101048.

Nouwen HJM, McNeill DP, Morrison DA (1982) Compassion: a reflection on the Christian life. New York: Doubleday.

Nussbaum MC (1996) Compassion: the basic social emotion. Social Philosophy and Policy, **13**, 27–58.

Nussbaum MC (2001) Upheavals in thought: the intelligence of emotions. Cambridge: Cambridge University Press.

Owain Hughes T (2013) The compassion quest. London: SPCK.

Pask E (2003) Moral agency in Nursing" Seeing value in the work and believing that I make a difference. Nursing Ethics, **10**(2), 165–174.

Pollock A (2004). NHS plc: the privatisation of our health care. Bath: Verso.

Randall F, Downie RS (2006) The philosophy of palliative care: critique and reconstruction. Oxford: Oxford University Press.

Riess H, Kelley JM, Bailey RW, Dunn EJ, Phillips M (2012) Empathy training for resident physicians: A randomized controlled trial of a neuroscience-informed curriculum. Journal of General Internal Medicine **27**(10), 1280–1286.

Rinpoche S, Gaffney P, Harvey A (2012) The Tibetan book of living & dying: the spiritual classic and international bestseller. San Francisco: Harper.

Rivett G (1998) From cradle to grave: 50 years of the NHS. London: King's Fund.

Sabo B (2008) Adverse psychological consequences: compassion fatigue, burnout and vicarious traumatization: are nurses who provide palliative and haematological cancer care vulnerable? Indian Journal of Palliative Care, **14**, 23–29.

Saslow LR et al. (2013) The social significance of spirituality: new perspectives on the compassion-altruism relationship. Psychology of Religion and Spirituality, **5**(3), 201–218.

Sasser CG, Pulchalski C.M. (2010) The humanistic clinician: traversing the science and art of health care. Journal of Pain and Symptom Management, **39**(5), 936–940.

Saunders C (1996) Into the valley of the shadow of death: a personal therapeutic journey. British Medical Journal, **7072**(313), 1599–1601.

Saunders C (2003) Watch with me: inspiration for a life in hospice care. London: Mortal Press.

Schantz M (2007) Compassion: a concept analysis. Nursing Forum **42**(2), 48–55.

Sears D (1998) Compassion for humanity in the Jewish tradition. Northvale, NJ: Jason Aronson.

Sevensky RL (1983) The religious foundations of health care: a conceptual approach. Journal of Medical Ethics, **9**, 165–169.

Singer T, Bolz M (eds) (2013) Compassion: bridging practice and science. Munich: Max Planck Society.

Smajdor A (2013) Should compassionate care be incentivised? Nursing Times, **109**, 49–50.

Svenaeus F (2014) The phenomenology of empathy in medicine: an introduction. Medicine, Health Care and Philosophy, **17**, 245–248.

Whitebrook M (2002) Compassion as a political virtue. Political Studies, **50**(3):529–544.

Wishart PM (2005) Conceptualising compassionate power. Spirituality and Health International, **6**(1), 33–38.

World Health Organisation (2002) Palliative care. http://www.who.int/cancer/palliative/definition/en/

Chapter 2

Janet Abrahm—Healing connections

Dr Janet Abrahm received her MD from the University of California at San Francisco (UCSF) in 1973, completed internship and residency at the Massachusetts General Hospital, and served as a chief resident at Moffitt Hospital of UCSF. She completed a fellowship in haematology/oncology at the hospital of the University of Pennsylvania and was a faculty member at the University of Pennsylvania School of Medicine from 1980 through 2000. Dr Abrahm built the first palliative care service at the Philadelphia VA Medical Center (PVAMC) and served for several years as chief of the medical service. In 1997 she secured the first NIH-funded Palliative Medicine Fellowship, which in 2003 was competitively renewed. In 2001, Dr Abrahm joined the Dana-Farber Cancer Institute (DFCI) to build what became the Adult Palliative Care Division of the Department of Psychosocial Oncology and Palliative Care at DFCI and Brigham and Women's Hospital. For ten years as board member and then officer of the American Academy of Hospice and Palliative Medicine, Dr Abrahm helped lead the field to specialty recognition and in 2006, she was named to the American Board of Internal Medicine's first test-writing committee for the hospice and palliative medicine board examination. She currently is a member of the Adult Palliative Care Division at DFCI and is a professor of medicine at Harvard Medical School.

Foundations in palliative and end-of-life care

My entry into the field of palliative care was a little different from that of many of my colleagues. I came to palliative medicine from my interest in pain and symptom management in cancer and haematology patients. I originally trained and practised haematology-oncology at the Hospital of the University of Pennsylvania and the PVAMC, both affiliates of the University of Pennsylvania School of Medicine. I practised haematology and oncology there for about 20 years. In addition to doing inpatient consultations, we established a comprehensive, patient-focused haematology-oncology clinic which was unlike most other clinics in that we were the primary outpatient care providers as well as the specialists. We developed an interdisciplinary team of doctors, nurses, nurse practitioners, physician assistants, social workers, clinical pharmacists, chaplains when available, and students—mainly nurse practitioner, clinical pharmacy, and health psychology students—essentially clinicians you would include today in a palliative care team. This was before palliative care began to be developed in the United States. At that time, I had very few drugs to treat the symptoms of my cancer and haematology patients. In the 1980s, the pain medications we used for outpatients were mainly NSAIDs, acetaminophen, immediate-release morphine, hydromorphone or oxycodone, a combination of oxycodone and aspirin (Percodan®) or oxycodone and acetaminophen (Percocet®). When I learned about methadone, I used it as my long-acting opioid. Most of the drug formulations we rely on today just did not exist. Drugs available to prevent or treat chemotherapy-induced nausea and vomiting were even less effective: lorazepam, prochlorperazine, and dexamethasone. Many of my younger patients could not handle the chemotherapy and some actually died because they would go to the Caribbean and try alternative therapies. I saw all the harm we could do with chemotherapy, even if we were curing people. Often we did not cure them or even prolong their lives. I became committed to doing whatever I could to prevent or control their symptoms. I became an avid reader of the literature on pain and symptom management and I applied it. I would say I was an 'early adopter' in today's terminology.

In the early 1990s, I was at a crossroads in the haematopoiesis research I had been doing; I realized that to stay in the field, I would need to learn the tools of molecular biology that were beginning to be applied. I recognized that I really preferred bringing disparate fields together, and taking a broad approach to solving problems rather than, as bench research required, delving deeply into a very specific aspect of a problem. I started to question what else I should do if I stopped working in haematopoiesis research. I realized that if I added a scholarly focus to my clinical interest in pain and symptom management, I could be a much-needed resource to our Haematology/Oncology Division at the University of Pennsylvania Hospital and the PVAMC.

In 1992, I took a sabbatical for three months with Dr Kathy Foley (see chapter 11) who then led the Pain Division of the Department of Neurology at Memorial Sloan Kettering Cancer Center (MSKCC). I had the good fortune to be there in the crucible with the pioneers that helped create the field of palliative care. I use the term *crucible* in the sense of it being an alchemical vessel that makes transformation possible. I spent three months there, almost 20 years out from medical school but a novice again, fascinated by the holistic approach that they were taking to assessing and treating cancer patients in pain and who suffered from delirium. Now, I recognize that while they called it a 'pain service', they approached patients who are suffering in the way we now define hospice and palliative care. I did not know enough to understand that then. The clinicians at MSKCC were developing the tools whereby we could assess people more comprehensively and the expertise to treat them much more effectively.

When I went back to my regular job, I got support so that I could spend more time using those tools in practice. I also decided that I needed to create a team like the one I had seen at MSKCC. I identified some resources to create such a team, led by a nurse practitioner, and including a chaplain, a social worker, and myself. I created a database to show the difference we made because the hospital administration was sceptical. The data demonstrated that across all domains of care for the patients we saw—even the oncology patients—our team alleviated patient symptoms, as well as social and spiritual distress. We published this data to show that a team like this in the VA system could really improve the patient's quality of life.

I found it fascinating to be educated by my team about psychological and spiritual needs and family dynamics, because as a haematologist/oncologist, I'd had no psychiatric training and no social worker or chaplain to teach me. Fortunately, I recruited an oncology nurse specialist, Mary Cooley, to work with me in our VA lung cancer clinic. She later became an oncology nurse practitioner and is now a senior NIH-funded nurse scientist based in the Cantor Center in Boston. Mary and I shared an office and we learned a great deal from each other. I learned that while I was expert in the medical models of how to treat lung cancer, Mary was an expert on oncology nursing models of how to help lung cancer patients and their families get through treatment, complications, and, eventually, their grief. I also learned a great deal from Mary's mentor, Dr Ruth McCorkle, who had created one of the largest databases on the symptoms of patients with lung cancer and from that, the international research resource, the Symptom Distress Scale. At Penn, when I began to focus my clinical work in what is now palliative care, I became involved with the research and educational efforts of Dr McCorkle and other oncology nursing professors in the University of Pennsylvania School of Nursing because at the time, medical oncologists at Penn were not doing symptom management research or educational programmes. I am delighted that we are still doing groundbreaking symptom management research together.

After I had been chief of the Haematology Oncology Division for about ten years, and had begun work in hospice and palliative care, I thought I needed a career move, and the chief of the medical service suggested I train with him towards becoming a chair of medicine at another facility. Unfortunately, he resigned a couple of weeks after I agreed to work with him and I became chief of the PVAMC Medical Service. I took that opportunity to create the same model of whole-person care that I had been delivering in my haematology/oncology clinic; we reorganized the entire medical service into an interdisciplinary collaborative service. It took about three years. At that point, someone sent me information on the Project on Death in America and an application to become a faculty scholar. For my proposed project, I thought end-of-life care would perfectly fit the disease management model then popular at Penn. We could work with our hospice to identify a group of patients who were hospice-eligible but not quite ready for hospice, use our disease management model to care for them, and enrol them into hospice when they were ready. I thought I would learn more about disease management and serve the Penn health system by being able to develop this programme for them. My application was successful, and I was chosen for the third cohort of the Project on Death in America faculty scholars. As part of that programme, I got to know Dr Susan Block and I learnt many things from her and the faculty she assembled, including how to be a change agent, but I still lacked mentors at Penn to help me develop my expertise in palliative care beyond pain and symptom management. Dr Block had taken the position of Division Chief of Psycho-Oncology and Palliative Care at DFCI in Boston, and was looking to bring in a palliative care colleague to lead the adult palliative care programme, so I thought that would be perfect because I had a huge gap in the psychosocial aspect of my clinical practice. As an oncologist, I thought I was well positioned to bring palliative care to Dana-Farber; I knew many of the Dana-Farber oncologists from my previous work. It is hard to learn locally when you are considered the expert and you don't have models around to learn from.

So I came to Dana-Farber and started the adult palliative care programme. I am pleased with my clinical growth in the psychological, social, and spiritual aspects of palliative care. The first edition of my book, *A Physician's Guide to Pain and Symptom Management in Cancer Patients*, came out in 2000 and in 2005, the second edition, which was much richer and more comprehensive. Through my career, I evolved from an oncologist and pain and symptom management expert into a true palliative medicine clinician. There were realms of experience that I was just fascinated by, particularly the spiritual and psychological issues affecting my patients' lives of which I had no understanding before I came to Boston. I wanted to open all those doors, learn about that, and see how I could be more helpful.

The latest evolution of my practice is working with Dr Eric Cassell around healing and suffering and working with my patients using hypnosis. I was trained in hypnosis long before we had the current analgesics and antiemetics and would use it for symptom management. That led me to learn more about imagery, and what people can do to heal themselves. So I have been helping people heal themselves using hypnosis for 20 years. I have been privileged to work with Eric as he wrote his book *The Nature of Healing: The Modern Practice of Medicine*, and I have had many conversations with him about how crucial function is to healing. Even as a medical student, I thought medicine's goal was to help people to function in a way that they wanted to. That is probably why I am attracted to the idea of compassion. For me, medicine was not only about curing disease. If I could find a way to restore my patients to a level of function so that they felt satisfied—that could also be my goal.

The compassionate practitioner

My understanding of compassion has evolved because you can only be as connected as you feel safe to be. It takes a long time to learn that being open helps you connect more and helps you feel safe. Becoming a professor in a very competitive academic environment such as Harvard holds an aspect of risk and you must have a willingness to take risks if you're going to connect. There are defences that you build up along the way. So becoming a compassionate practitioner is essentially about the presence of one human to another. I remember working in the county hospitals with alcoholics and drug addicts and people who had really had a rough life. I remember feeling very compassionate towards them. For whatever reason, this was the life they were leading, and I was there to help them get back to a life in which they could have some meaning and function and not suffer so much. I remember even back then not being angry when they kept getting readmitted. My colleagues were angry. I just had a different standard.

For me, compassion is not related to faith or religious practice. I was nominally raised in the Jewish faith. Through my teenage years, I did all the usual things, going to temple on the high holidays and becoming educated in my faith. Something about medical school, though, the reality of that cadaver, the immediacy of life and death—since my first year of medical school I haven't felt the need for a connection to a higher being. I do feel the need for connection and I would consider myself spiritual because I feel very connected. If I am not connected I am not happy. I feel being compassionate is being connected, caring, but also having enough self-awareness so that I am still a professional. Empathy always feels a little condescending to me. I can empathize with your situation but I am not connected to it. For me, empathy has too much of the intellectual about it. Compassion is often seen in a Buddhist context. I am not a Buddhist but I have done a lot of reading in that area and I do mindfulness meditation. Compassion is a human connection, often non-verbal, which can be used therapeutically. If you cannot connect, you should ask yourself why not, what is the problem? Eric Cassell has taught me that the most healing aspect of what we do is connecting and not leaving a person alone in his or her suffering. When I go in there as a physician bringing all the Western medical knowledge, I really want to develop trust. If I am compassionate, it feels as though I am open and you can sense that you can say anything you need to tell me. Professionally, that is the most important thing that can happen in a clinical relationship—that people tell you about their suffering and things that are bothering them. If they trust you with that you can be a really helpful clinician to them.

I find Henri Nouwen's definition interesting. I agree with the idea of 'sharing in brokenness, entering into places of pain'—all of that. 'Going where it hurts' makes me question how I can best help this person heal. ('Heal', after all is etymologically cognate with 'whole') (Nouwen et al. 1982: 4). I have to know where they hurt to help them heal. I need to be able to hold the hurt—*their* hurt, of course, not our hurt, but I have to help them contain it, sometimes share it, sometimes just understand it, explore it, put light on it. If you have compassion there is no barrier. Empathy gets in the way of that a little for me—it is more distant.

I model compassion to teach it to our physicians, rather than doing didactic teaching. We have students and residents on clinical rotations so, for example, whenever I use hypnosis with a patient, I model that form of connection. Whenever they notice that a patient and I have made a special connection, we discuss what happened, what I was doing to make it happen, and, if I used hypnosis, I explain how that helped. If they are open to it, I suggest to them that this is the kind of training you need in medicine. I try to pique an interest in learning hypnosis and mindfulness in anyone who seems to connect naturally or to appreciate what I was doing and who wants to learn how to do it themselves.

I feel deeply that those who enter the healing professions are compassionate, and, as Rachel Naomi Remen (http://www.rachelremen.com) describes, we all have the *flame*. She teaches the first-year medical students that you need to protect the flame because so much threatens it, particularly in medical school—you could call that flame 'compassion'. What we have to do is put them in touch with that flame and teach them how to maintain and protect the compassion that they went into medicine with, to avoid being overwhelmed. I think we have to help students understand that being open is the safest way to be and also teach them techniques such as hypnosis and mindfulness that will help them be open. They can bring these tools to their clinical encounters. In psychiatry, they teach a concept called 'observing presence'. Perhaps developing an observing presence, supported by preceptors working at different clinical levels to help with connection, and teaching students ways to keep that connection going would be useful. We can show them that as they grow in technical expertise, they can also grow in their ability to connect without losing that flame, how to foster it and grow in it and use it as they do all their other clinical skills. Having people like Rachel Naomi Remen in medical school is as valuable as all the microbiologists and geneticists are. I definitely think education and pedagogy has a great place in fostering a compassionate graduating class or a future compassionate clinician.

A case exemplar

I can tell you about a patient with sickle cell disease whom I looked after for many years. I did not know why I resonated with people with chronic pain until I became a faculty scholar and we were doing exercises about how you came to palliative care. Everybody but me talked about end-of-life care. I talked about having a back injury as an intern and having severe pain. I did not need surgery but I had many years where I would be unable to work for a week or two, to the point where I had to be wheeled out of the office by chair to the car because I pushed it too far and could not move anymore. That was just my life. It was subconscious, I am sure, but obviously I would have compassion for patients with sickle cell disease. When I met him, he was a man in his 30s, suffering all the ravages of the disease: enormous liver, no spleen, leg ulcers—but with enormous dignity. He was a fabulous man. He was trying to write his memoirs and always brought this huge file of papers with him. He was a role model for his nephews and nieces; he had no children of his own. Now we have drugs and transfusions that can ameliorate symptoms but this was long before we had any treatments that addressed sickle crises. When I first met him, I had immediate compassion for him. Working with him I learned to recognize what chronic pain looked like. When he first came in he would not move at all. I knew he was telling me the truth that he was in pain. I had to fight for him all the time to get the drugs he needed, because nobody would give drugs to sickle cell patients. Clinicians thought sickle cell patients were drug-seeking because they (the clinicians) did not know what chronic pain looked like. He never had any of the signs of acute pain, his pulse and blood pressure were normal, and he was not crying out—this is long before pain became the fifth clinical sign—so the nurses would not give him analgesia. As his pain crises abated, he became more mobile, would interact with people, and became his usual self a day or so before he was discharged. You would think I would have recognized myself immediately in his story, but I didn't. I knew I was in severe pain, and was cranky when my back went out and I could not move, but I didn't have a lot of self-insight and I was so busy denying my disability that I didn't recognize the similarities in our situations until many years later. What I saw in him, though, I could see, in my cancer patients. I learnt from the Brief Pain Inventory (http://www.mdanderson.org) to ask my patients questions about function, and as we would treat the pain, these people would become cheerful, helpful, and cooperative. They could tolerate the test they needed to get their diagnosis—they could function again. Compassion was the beginning because without compassion there would have been no trust and I would not have believed him. He was from a different culture, a different race, different socio-economic level—different everything. But his dignity and patience in his suffering was enormous. When I learnt hypnosis, I said to him, 'You have been doing this your whole life.' He said, 'Well, how else do you think I get through this? I just take my mind away.' So he became my teacher and I became his doctor and his friend, and as we went through the years together, I would come back from the VA and see him at the hospital. When he finally died, his family sent a car to take me to the funeral because they thought it was not safe in their neighbourhood and they wanted to be sure that I did not drive. They put me in the front pew of the church. I honoured him as a patriarch and mentor for his family and loved ones, despite all his illness and suffering. I have a little plaque he gave me one time which I still keep. He looked after me; we looked after each other. If I did anything here, it was that in the depth of his despair, I was able to help him see his power, his reach, and the enormous love there was for him. I helped him connect at times when he couldn't by relieving some of his physical suffering and also reminding him *who he was.* That is what I felt my compassion was doing for him. I have not thought of this in a while so I am glad to think of him again.

Fostering sustainable compassion

I think I relate to the controversy regarding the over-professionalization of palliative care because, thanks to support from the Project on Death in America, I became both an academic palliative care clinician and a hospice medical director when academic palliative care was just beginning. I remember the conversations I had with my hospice nursing colleagues as we discovered different ways of showing that we cared for patients. As an academic palliative care physician, I didn't think it was right to simply treat a symptom and not give any thought to its cause. As a hospice medical director, I didn't think it was right not to give any thought to the burden of clinical tests just to figure out what the cause was. We found that there was plenty of room for compromise on both sides, and that the evidence base does not have to be an enemy of compassion; it can be a servitor of compassion. We arrived at a middle ground where we weighed the burden versus the benefit of discovering a cause, in case a technological solution would provide more sustained relief. For example, if someone in a hospice programme has two to three months to live and they are hypercal-caemic, of course you would treat them to restore function as much as possible. They may become hypercalcaemic at the very end of their life, but what should one do about earlier instances in their final illness when they still have so much to do in those months? If they had a large pleural effusion that could be drained and that could perhaps reduce the need for opioids, then why would you not do that? Those are simple examples. That has been the kind of tension I have seen—even in my hospice team. The decision on the degree of intervention should be based on the goals of this patient. What does it take to help them function in their spiritual, psychological, social, and physical realms? How do we craft a plan weighing the burdens and benefits of all of the things, both diagnostic and therapeutic, that we can do? How do we individualize that for you now and in the future? How do we make an acceptable plan of medical care that does not overtreat or immerse you in that treatment? It takes skill, compassion, and a close connection. It takes a very sophisticated, professional team assessment to balance the different goals as they change.

Palliative care holds that changing space, because we are the ones who help people move from trying to prolong their lives with technological advances to understanding that those now have become more of a burden than a benefit for them. I don't know if all hospice staff understand the difficulties of holding that space because they may not have much experience with that transition; they may see themselves as ministering and helping people who have already made the decision to transfer to hospice. They don't have to be in conflict. But what if hospice finances changed so that they could enrol people on supportive treatments such as total parenteral nutrition, knowing that they had a six-month prognosis, using it when it helped them meet their goals, and then helping them wean off when it no longer did, and in the process helping patients find meaning and purpose beyond prolonging their lives? If the financial arrangements were such that we were able to give the technical treatments when they were useful and not when they were not within a context of care that employed palliative hospice care techniques—that would help primary care and specialist practitioners not have to make the terrible choices we are asking them to make now. Then, we would be better able to help the family to feel successful in bringing their loved one to the best possible end of life. This should be a collaborative effort, if we could only each give a bit and work better together. It comes back to trust.

I think the way to help medical students prevent burnout has to do with a realistic counselling approach—helping them gain self-insight, helping them try to figure out what it means to them to be successful in life, what is valuable to them, what is important, and to let them know they'll need to re-evaluate frequently. I have always had five-year plans. I re-evaluated what I was doing every five years: if it was still good for another five years, fine, and if not, I would seek other options. Asking myself, 'Am I happy?' and changing jobs if the answer was 'No!' was an expectation for me and not a failure. As the world changes, I change; my needs change. So I should pay attention!

The key to helping medical students keep their compassion is to teach them self-compassion, which took me years to learn, and I am still learning it. Serious insight and training in self-compassion is easy to say and hard to do for most professions. If you have that kind of compassion it is easier for you to have compassion for patients and colleagues. Without it, you can still have compassion for patients but you risk burning out or having compassion fatigue because you don't know how to hold the pain and grief, or find the support you need. You need to find a way to connect into your compassion, maybe through meditation or deep hypnosis. However you get it, *more power to you!*

Commentary

Two themes stand out from this chapter by Janet Abrahm—connection and healing. Both would seem to be important components in understanding the shape of palliative and hospice care in America today. The Open Society Institute (http://www.soros.org) Project on Death in America (PDIA) provided the research and scholarship designed to transform the culture and practice of care for dying people. Through grant aid in priority areas, the creation of faculty scholars to effect institutional change, economic and legislative engagement and philanthropic endeavour, PDIA sought to enhance capacity and embed palliative care into institutions to 'facilitate the compassionate care of the dying' (Aulino & Foley 2001: 492). Of note, the project made the point that health care systems needed to connect more cohesively to the public so their complex discourse about death could be heard and clear messages about death and dying in society offered. The skills that are required to achieve this, such as attentive listening, attunement to patient narrative, and self-reflection have been called for through innovative curricula which seek a holistic rather than dualistic approach to learning (Boudreau, Cassell, & Fuks 2007).

The US distinction between *palliative* care (which is an extra layer of support for patients at any stage of a life-limiting illness) and *hospice* care (which is limited to patients with a life expectancy of about six months if the disease takes its usual course) is an important one. In countries where palliative care and hospice care are seen interchangeably, the discussion about the meaning and impact of what hospice means may be less evident. Transition simply happens, perhaps clouded under the guise of seamless care. In the US model, careful conversations about the cessation of life-prolonging treatment are generally needed for access to hospice care, though there are so-called open-access hospices. Part of the problem is financial: the hospice programmes in the US are reimbursed to approximately $160 per day to pay for all the personnel, medical equipment, drugs, and oxygen a patient needs. Only the largest hospice programmes can offer the full range of palliative therapies, such as radiation therapy to painful bony metastases. One might consider that this potentially opens a more honest and appropriate dialogue with the patient and family about living and dying well. What it does require is the integrity and dedication of the clinician to lead gently on the right path. That needs a healing connection to have been made so that trust, faith, and a spirit of openness can be established. And the basis of that healing connection speaks to the essence of a compassionate practitioner.

The relationship between healing and suffering at end of life has been a topic of academic exploration. The writing of Balfour Mount and Michael Kearney (2003), Rachel Naomi Remen (2006, 2008, 2013), and Eric Cassell (2014) in particular are examples of the call from and by clinicians to examine what we mean by some of the concepts which underpin clinical practice but which, perhaps, have not been unpacked. A noteworthy paper by Thomas Egnew (2005) sought to understand the meaning of healing through a series of interviews with seven eminent 'allopathic' physicians, including Eric Cassell, Elizabeth Kubler-Ross, Carl Hammerschlag, and Cicely Saunders. Healing was defined in terms of wholeness, narrative, and spirit with a confluence of subthemes, including transcendence, meaning, and reconciliation. In this paper, Hammerschlag defines a healer as one 'who is going to help you make those connections between each other and everything around you' (p. 257). The call made here by Janet Abrahm is that this is not just between clinician and patient, but between teacher and student so that the eloquently described *flame* which has been ignited in the soul of the neophyte learner can be nurtured and tended by the adept practitioner to set them on a career path which is both healing and sustaining. Recognizing that need stems from a place of compassion and wisdom within expert practice and commitment to a compassionate way of being.

Reflections for practice

- Consider what the flame as described here means to you and how that can be nurtured to support and guide you in your practice and your career in palliative and end-of-life care.

- What do you understand by Janet Abrahm's suggestion that evidence can be the 'servitor of compassion'? How do you see that relationship?

- In what way can you as a palliative care practitioner 'hold the space' for your patient or client in their transitions between the pathways of health care?

Further reading

Aulino F, Foley K (2001) The Project on Death in America. Journal of the Royal Society of Medicine, **94**, 492–495.

Boudreau JD, Cassell EJ, Fuks A (2007) A healing curriculum. Medical Education, **41**, 1193–1201.

Cassell E (2004) The nature of suffering and the goals of medicine (2nd ed.). Oxford: Oxford University Press.

Cassell E (2014) The nature of healing: the modern practice of medicine. Oxford: Oxford University Press.

Egnew TR (2005) The meaning of healing: transcending suffering. Annals of Family Medicine, **3**(3), 255–262.

Mount B, Kearney M (2003) Healing and palliative care: charting our way forward. Palliative Medicine, **17**, 657–658.

Nouwen HJM, McNeill DP, Morrison DA (1982) Compassion: a reflection on the Christian life. New York: Doubleday.

Rabow MW, Carrie NE, Remen RN (2013) Repression of personal values and qualities in medical education. Family Medicine, **45**(1), 13–18.

Remen RN (2001) My grandfather's blessings: stories of strength, refuge and belonging. New York: Riverhead.

Remen RN (2006) Kitchen table wisdom. New York: Riverhead.

Remen RN (2008) Practicing a medicine of the whole person: an opportunity for healing. Hematology/Oncology Clinics of North America, **22**(4), 767–773.

Chapter 3

Mary Baines— Understanding pity

Mary Baines trained with Cicely Saunders at St Thomas's Hospital in London. After qualification, she worked for ten years as a general practitioner before joining the staff at St Christopher's Hospice a few months after it opened. Two years later, she was involved in setting up the first hospice home care service, offering symptom control and support to terminally ill patients and their families.

Her seminal research on the pharmacological management of patients with inoperable intestinal obstruction has been published widely. She has written extensively including chapters in four Oxford textbooks and has presented at numerous international conferences, including giving the first plenary lecture on palliative care at the Union for International Cancer Control UICC conference in New Delhi in 1994. Her work in the field of palliative care has been acknowledged with the award of an OBE and an honorary doctorate at the University of Greenwich. On her retirement, she was appointed emeritus consultant at St Christopher's Hospice, Sydenham.

Foundations in palliative and end-of-life care

I was a medical student with Cicely Saunders and that goes right back. I met Cicely in 1954, having done my pre-med at Cambridge. We then had to come to London for the clinical course. So Cicely and I were medical students, exact contemporaries—although she was much older than me. We qualified in the same year 1957. I got married, went into general practice part-time, and I was very happily settled in that. Cicely, as people know, was motivated by her calling to improve the care of the dying. She went on to study the control of pain and she collected a group around her who shared her vision. In 1964 she made an appeal on the BBC for money to build a hospice. I happened to hear this and sent her £3, which is more than it is now; I became a friend of St Christopher's and went to the opening in July 1967. Soon after that I had a nice letter from Cicely asking if I would like to come and see around St Christopher's as a local GP. Of course, that wasn't the real reason. She wanted me to join her on the staff.

I said no at first. I was happy as a part-time GP; we had three small children. And yet I thought about it, talked it over with medical friends who thought it was professional suicide. But I joined her. Why did I join her? Because I thought it was the right thing to do, and I guess because of the medical excitement of making a difference in a completely new branch of medicine. I joined her in April 1968, so I have been a hospice doctor since then but in an honorary capacity since I retired at 70.

St Christopher's was not the first hospice, but it was the first modern hospice, the first hospice that combined teaching and research with clinical care. In the early days, there were fewer staff and more patients than there are now. There are now 48 patients but when we opened the unit it was 54—we went up to 62 and then down to 48. We had considerably fewer medical staff but still did regular ward rounds. From the beginning, the documentation covered psychological, social, and spiritual factors as well as purely physical ones. The patient population was different; we had a number of patients who stayed there for considerably longer than they would nowadays.

In 1969, I was involved in starting the first home care service. A women in her 50s with bone metastasis from breast cancer surprised Cicely by saying something like 'Thank you very much for all you have done for me at St Christopher's, and I am grateful that my pain is now relieved, but actually I want to go home.' This threw Cicely badly because people did not go home. They liked it at St Christopher's and were grateful for the care and stayed until they died. I was given the job of arranging her discharge. I contacted the GP, discussed the woman's medication, gave her a good supply of the drugs she needed which included a moderate dose of diamorphine, and duly she went home. Ten or eleven days later, we got a call from her husband to say she was in agony and please could she come back. We found out that her GP had visited her, had thought we were turning his patient into a drug addict, so tailored down the diamorphine—with the result of course that the pain came back. It was easy to control her pain, we just put her back on the drug she was having previously. It's a sad story because she never went home again. She lost her nerve, and stayed in St Christopher's until she died. It was following this episode that Cicely said 'We must start home care now.' She did not ask us; she told us what to do. I am just grateful how we started the service. Barbara McNulty, a nurse, and I spent some months going around GPs and district nurses in the community to say 'Do you want a hospice service at home, and if so, what shape do you want it to be?' The answer came back: Yes, they did want help at home, particularly pain and symptom control and counselling in its broadest sense. They wanted to remain in charge of patients at home; the district nurses wanted to continue the practical nursing that was needed. So that is how it was set up. It is what the community wanted.

Fairly quickly we had 80 patients, which went on for quite a time and what I think caused it to expand was the development of palliative care services in our hospitals. Part of discharge planning for people with advanced disease was to refer to a hospice home care service. Now the numbers under the care of St Christopher's home care service is around 800—and 48 beds. So for me, the home care service is the most important part of what we offer.

Just over a year ago, the Cicely Saunders Institute at Kings College Hospital put on a concert to celebrate the development of home care and to mark my 80th birthday. The event was also to celebrate the development of palliative home care, and I invited three of the original GPs from 1969 to attend. One of them said to me, 'Mary, it needed humility on both sides, we learnt together'— and that is where I think it fitted in. The second service, at St Joseph's Hospice in Hackney, was different and the palliative care team did everything. I have no doubt at all that they had a good service for patients, but for me it was not the right model. Why would the GP and district nurse want to hand over somebody they had been involved with for some time to palliative care when they were dying? I didn't think it was right.

Cicely taught people like me that our job was twofold—one was to look after the patients on the wards and later the patients at home, to the best of our ability. That's fairly obvious. The second was to change the world's view of dying. It was a pretty ambitious aim for a small unit in South London. The important thing is that we can tell people what palliative care involves—managing the 'total pain' as Cicely called it. What we must never, ever do is to tell people where or how to do it. They have to work that out themselves within their own resources. There have been a few disasters where people have gone out and told people how to do it. We have no right to do that; we are not the right people.

When I arrived Cicely gave me a single sheet of A4 folded, and she said, 'Mary, this is symptom control, go and put it into practice and you will be OK.' We then went on writing and researching, my own research was into the management of malignant bowel obstruction. That was the first paper in 1984. The body of knowledge at St Christopher's increased from one single sheet of A4 to the Oxford textbooks and all the things that came after—which is marvellous. It is an incredible story, which has gone around the world!

The compassionate practitioner

I have read the Henri Nouwen definition that is about entering into the hurt of others, into their places of pain. I actually prefer the one from the *Concise Oxford Dictionary*, which describes compassion as 'Pity, inclining one to help'. In other words, compassion is an emotion leading to the probability of action. I like the two together—that it is an experience of entering into the hurt of others that very often will lead one to help. This definition helps doctors and nurses who are basically practical people.

This said, I have my doubts as to whether a deep compassion is necessary in all medical practice for it takes time and special energy to enter into the hurts of others. This became clear to me about three years ago when my husband had a succession of hospital admissions and only one doctor, on one occasion, asked him a very simple question: 'What did you do?' He showed an interest in my husband as a person. This was pleasant but not necessary. My husband had excellent care from doctors who were kind, competent, and good at their jobs. Perhaps in many branches of medicine we need kind technicians.

However, in palliative care and older person care, patients have serious life-threatening or disabling conditions. They do need staff able to enter into their suffering and bring practical and emotional support. This is especially necessary in doctors and nurses because they are involved all the time. Social workers are needed to care for patients and families with complicated problems and to teach us how to manage the rest.

It is hard to say if we have lost compassion in palliative care. I still get many people who contact me to tell me about a relative or friend who was in a hospice or was cared for at home by a hospice team and the health care professionals really cared; nothing was too much trouble—that sort of thing. But I do think that the push for nurses to get further qualifications is a bit of a challenge as is the computerization of all records. Sometimes it seems that doctors and nurses spend more time at a computer screen than they do talking or just sitting with patients.

A case exemplar

I have thought about two. They are quite short. What I decided to focus on were situations when compassion was difficult, often extremely difficult. I have to remind myself that although we are told that we should love our neighbours, we are not told that we should like our neighbours. Some of the people we look after we do not like very much.

In the first case the patient was in her 40s and she had multiple sclerosis. She was with us for many months, for at that time we took people for considerably longer than now. I can't remember where she came from, probably a hospital. Her husband was now living with another woman and we were told very firmly that we were not to inform her of this because she did not know. The staff all knew and many people were quite angry with him. There was considerable deceit needed when she talked to us about her devoted husband. I felt that he did not tell her to save her suffering but it was not a situation where it was particularly easy to be compassionate towards him. Yet that poor man had been on his own. She had been ill for a long time with a slowly progressive illness. The team struggled with this, trying to understand and enter into the hurt of this man. Fortunately for him, it was before we had mobile phones. For otherwise the patient might have rung up and found the other woman answering! Real compassion, when you don't like or approve of the person, is a difficult one.

Eventually the patient died and we lost touch with the man. But, to give him credit, he came up every few days to visit his wife, sat with her and that brought her comfort. So, maybe, he did the best thing. I don't know!

My other case is recent and is about a neighbour of mine, a widower of 89 who lived on his own. He had developed a deep vein thrombosis and investigations showed a large clot in the right atrium. The hospital doctors expected him to throw off a large pulmonary embolus. He had refused anticoagulants and said that he wanted to die and was determined to stay at home, with no interference. He refused the GP's offer to contact the hospice home care team.

The thing I found difficult in this situation is when he said to me, 'If you live to 89 and see all that I have seen, you would know that there is no God.' We all find it hard when patients aggressively challenge our deeply held beliefs. But it is helpful to remember that compassion—pity plus action—does not require us to like or agree with everyone we care for. I was so grateful when the elderly man died peacefully at home and did not need emergency drugs, which the hospice team would have organized but which he refused.

When our natural instinct is to dislike someone, we find it difficult to be compassionate. This was true for me with the husband who was deceiving his wife and the elderly neighbour. We still care but it isn't easy. I have often talked about this and there have been a few times when I have thought, 'I have nothing to give of myself to this patient; I am done in today. So I will for now simply be a doctor.' I would examine patients, prescribe the necessary drugs, but would not get involved in deeper emotional things because I hadn't got it to give. If a patient wanted to start that sort of conversation, I would alert a colleague. As doctors and nurses involved in end-of-life care, we need to know when to say no.

Fostering sustainable compassion

I think that choosing the right staff is the most important factor if you want to build a compassionate team. This is boasting but most of the original leaders in palliative care were trained at St Christopher's. We didn't advertise. People just came to us. Many people were inspired by the Christian foundation, and we looked at the whole person, not just at the number of papers he or she had written. We can be faulted on our way of choosing people but what we cannot be faulted on is the calibre of those people who came out, for we looked for compassion in them. I don't know if compassion can be taught in a lecture but there is no doubt that it can be modelled; it is an apprenticeship thing. Staff in training need to go on ward rounds where emotional and spiritual issues are brought up. But this must be done in non-threatening ways with open questions such as 'What is the worst thing about all this?'

My daughter is a psychiatrist and in her three years training she spent six months in general practice. This included attending GP training days and on one occasion there was a lecture on communication skills. She came back and said, 'Mum, it was dreadful, they teach you to look as if you care when you don't.'

I would like to say one other thing. I looked up references in the New Testament to where Jesus was 'moved with compassion' and I found ten. But in almost every place the quotation continues as 'He was moved with compassion *and* . . .' It wasn't just that he felt sorry for the person; his compassion led to action. This leads me back to my *Concise Oxford Dictionary* definition of compassion as 'pity, inclining one to help'. Looking at the worldwide spread of palliative care, it is very often Christians who have started the work. The Christian foundation of hospice must not be forgotten.

Commentary

Mary Baines offers the sagacity of founder spirit. Having grown with the modern hospice movement, she embraces that through her thorough explication of the craft of palliative medicine. Moreover, she echoes the Christian foundational thinking that inspired Cicely Saunders to want to care in this different way for those who were dying. The idea of compassion as pity, cited in her chosen definition, is a complex one and often challenged in theoretical literature. Either compassion and pity are one and the same (often cited by philosophers and ethicists) or differ by virtue of the fact that you can feel pity for someone but not be motivated to do anything about it (Crisp 2008). Feldman's (2005) description of a patient's experience of receiving pity from friends and relatives as 'longing for the visiting hour to be over so they could leave'(p. 50) would seem contrary to the engagement and being present to suffering that compassion evokes. In the two short clinical cases offered, Mary Baines shares one of the most challenging aspects of the compassionate response: when the person in need of compassion is someone we may dislike. In *The Hiding Place* Corrie Ten Boom describes her experience of coming face-to-face with an ex-guard from the Ravensbrück concentration camp many years after she was incarcerated for hiding Jews in her home in World War II. In that moment, she could only feel anger and hurt. Carr (1999) proposes that 'compassion involves a consideration of other people's values, beliefs, needs and wants in term of which their suffering can be understood and hence be shared' (p. 411). Ten Boom's ability to embrace that sense of shared suffering enabled her to reach out and take the hand of this man, despite her own antipathy. When patients and families are receptive to our care, it is certainly easier to engage with them meaningfully. It is considerably more difficult when not. There are certain times when the competent and efficient clinician embodies the reality of compassionate medicine. In the same clinical situation, the ability to engender a compassionate milieu may vary, depending on personal resources, patient and family response, and clinical context (Fernando & Considine 2013). In this sense, the ability to be compassionate to self as well as others and understand the limitations of constant caregiving is an essential component for palliative care practice.

Reflections for practice

◆ Consider the idea of compassion in the context of pity. How might you discriminate between them?

◆ What are the factors that you consider may impinge on your ability to be a compassionate practitioner in the first case offered in this chapter?

◆ It is argued that sometimes you have 'nothing left to give' and need to simply be a clinician. How does that influence your understanding of compassionate care?

Further reading

Carr B (1999) Pity and compassion as social virtues. Philosophy, 3, 411–429.

Crisp R (2008) Compassion and beyond. Ethical Theory, Morality and Practice, 11, 233–246.

Feldman C (2005) Compassion: listening to the cries of the world. Berkeley, CA: Rodmell.

Fernando AT, Consedine NS (2013) Beyond compassion fatigue: the transactional model of physician compassion. Journal of Pain and Symptom Management. http://dx.doi.org/10.1016/j.jpainsymman.2013.09.014

Fowler FG, Fowler HG (1964) The concise Oxford dictionary of current English. Oxford: Oxford University Press.

Ten Boom C, Sherill J, Sherill E (1984) The hiding place. London: Bantam.

Chapter 4

Ira Byock—Service

Ira Byock, MD, is a leading palliative care physician, author, and public advocate for improving care through the end of life. He is executive director and chief medical officer for the Institute for Human Caring of Providence Health and Services, CA. He is also Professor of Medicine and Community and Family Medicine at the Geisel School of Medicine at Dartmouth and served as Director of Palliative Medicine at Dartmouth-Hitchcock Medical Center in Lebanon, New Hampshire, from 2003 through July 2013. During the 1990s he was a co-founder and principal investigator for the Missoula Demonstration Project, a community-based organization in Montana dedicated to the research and transformation of end-of-life experience locally, as a demonstration of what is possible nationally. He also served as Director for Promoting Excellence in End-of-Life Care, a national grant programme of the Robert Wood Johnson Foundation.

Dr Byock has authored numerous articles on the ethics and practice of hospice, palliative, and end-of-life care, including *Dying Well* (1997), *The Four Things That Matter Most* (2004), and his most recent book, *The Best Care Possible* (2012), that tackles the crisis surrounding serious illness and dying in America.

As a consistent advocate for the voice and rights of dying patients and their families, he has been a featured guest on numerous US television and radio programmes and received many awards and commendations for this work. He is also a past president (1997) of the American Academy of Hospice and Palliative Medicine.

Foundations in palliative and end-of-life care

I was going to be a rural family practitioner. That is what I went to medical school to do and, frankly, that is what I thought I was going to do all through school and my post-residency training. During my residency training, I became involved in developing a fledging hospice programme to meet the unmet needs of a county hospital which served as a safety net hospital for the public of the central valley of California and it just got under my skin. This was not because of the suffering we were able to alleviate, but because of the sense of well-being I sometimes witnessed in people who were dying or whose loved ones were dying. That was surprising to me. There were a lot of questions in my mind: what does well-being look like towards the end of life? How do we foster that? Why is it that in some people we can barely alleviate suffering, and in others there is clearly a sense of well-being? So I got very involved and that has remained my focus through the years.

In the 1980s, it was not possible to make a living as a physician in hospice care in America, and in residency I become equally enamoured with emergency medicine. I became board-certified in emergency medicine and that is what I did for about 15 years. Along the way, wherever I was living, I was also a hospice medical director. Gradually, there grew to be more professional opportunities in palliative care as collectively—I and a number of other leading physicians—all contributed to its maturation. I was asked to lead a national grant and technical assistance project organized by the Robert Wood Johnson Foundation called Promoting Excellence in End-of-Life Care. It was an honour to do so. I was able to direct the programme from the town of Missoula, Montana, and developed a national office for the initiative based at the University of Montana. I had just over nine fabulous years directing that project. At the end of that, I went on to direct one of the many programmes that we had supported and became the director of palliative medicine at Dartmouth-Hitchcock Medical Center and at Dartmouth's Geisel School of Medicine in Dartmouth, New Hampshire. I have just left that position to move to Los Angeles where I hope to support them in their next level of clinical transformation in palliative care.

The compassionate practitioner

I like Henri Nouwen's description of compassion; his work is wonderful but I don't think it actually constitutes a definition. I think a definition has a different construct and format to it. Nor do I think it is Christian any more than Buddhist any more than it is Jewish.

For me, compassion is the experience of feeling the emotions and experience of the other, when the other is suffering. Compassion is a subset of empathy. Empathy is a sense of atonement (*at-one-ment*) and vicarious experience of the emotional state of the other. Compassion is empathy when the other person is suffering.

It is not just about palliative care, although I think palliative care has been instrumental in this. It is about taking the best care we can of another person, bringing all of our professional expertise, our knowledge base, our skill set, but as one person to another—where one has trained and committed to serve and the other is in need. It is not about us as caregivers or professionals. It is always about the other person.

Compassion is about going back to the best of one's mind or heart and just being as fully present with the other person as you can be authentically. In one sense, it starts with compassion being a natural state. The medical profession, and medical training in particular, approach seriously ill people through the lens of the medical model. It is a problem-based model. People come to doctors with problems; we assess them by making problem lists and then for every problem under the list create subjective and objective information, an assessment and a plan. As useful as that is, problem-based medicine does not capture the experience of illness. Ultimately illness is not medical; it is fundamentally personal. Serious illness carries both the large potential for suffering as well as the potential for the sense of well-being—which nobody talks about.

When you are actually with people you would need to be blind not to see it. It is so interesting that our language and our medical model and teaching almost keep us from seeing well-being, even when it is right in front of us. There is the human capacity for well-being, even as we are dying. The first book I wrote is titled, *Dying Well: Peace and Possibilities at the End of Life*. I chose 'well' really carefully. The word *well* is not just not an adverb describing the process or experience of dying; it is also an adjective describing the person who is dying. A person can be dying and be well. That for me is the highest therapeutic outcome I could hope for.

People bring different language to what I think is the same thing around compassion. Joan Halifax for example has developed a mnemonic around cultivating compassion (G.R.A.C.E.). It is recently published in the *Journal of Nursing Education and Practice* (Halifax 2014) so it speaks very much to a nursing audience. It would not be the particular language I would choose, but it is great work.

My approach entails a practice which I call therapeutic imagination. I try to imagine what it is like to be the patient, and listen to the patient's story as if I were the storyteller, try to see the world metaphorically as if I were looking through the person's eyes. I sometimes talk about employing receptive imagination with the goal of coming into imaginative alignment with the ill person. It requires a certain amount of centring; just taking a breath or two and just letting go, grounding, being present, letting go of other stuff I need to do and all that, but also letting go of my own stuff as far as possible, a sort of emptying. I first learned meditation through a Buddhist and Hindu tradition—now we call it mindfulness. That is an ongoing practice for me. I don't have a particular religious discipline: I was raised Jewish, but I see myself as a Jewish guy with a world view which is certainly more Buddhist in outlook. I meditate every day, but when I am with a patient I will just take a breath and just sort of let go. Psychiatry suggests that we are like tuning forks. If you are in a room with a patient, and you were not depressed going into the room but become depressed in the room, it is a good chance that the patient is depressed. If you know yourself well enough, it is a pretty useful diagnostic tool. This is where compassion comes in, because you have to be willing to feel the pain, or some degree of it. I don't want to overstate this, but the extent that I can be in therapeutic alignment is important—the pain the patient is feeling pangs in my chest as well. I have to just breathe and keep my heart open, to not close up and shrink and not turn away. Looking through his or her eyes, I can question whether there is something still to be achieved within their world views, their values, and their needs, which would not just alleviate suffering but move them towards a sense of well-being. That exercise often results in a therapeutic approach that could not be generated through a solely problem-based approach.

It is our presumption and our projections that limit people's ability to experience or talk about a sense of well-being. We, as clinicians, never ask about it. We direct their attention back to their problems and their distress. That is not entirely wrong, it is just not complete. It bothers me that this is not talked about much within palliative care. I am sort of an outlier who keeps bringing it up, sometimes to the discomfort of my colleagues. They think I am being romantic: 'Oh, Ira, you are talking about well-being and we are dealing with suffering.' Frankly I reject the criticism. I believe the omission of any discourse around well-being is anti-intellectual; it is avoiding the anthropology and nature of the human experience—the phenomenology of illness, if you will.

I think the professions outside medicine get this. Medical training and the practice of medicine today is really disease diagnosis and treatment system and that is what we teach, that is what we practice, that is what we pay for, and that is what we chart. It is all diagnosis and treatment and it keeps us from seeing well-being. Of course not every dying person experiences a sense of well-being by any means, but I believe it occurs more often than we recognize. At some point it is necessary to see medical problems within the larger context of one's life. Unfortunately, because we do not name it, the realization that 'this is my life!' often arises out of frustration for patients. They go to the doctor and they keep being offered more treatments. At some point it dawns on them that this is their life and medical interventions are constricting their personal time and energy which is waning. In every lecture I give, I make the point that the fundamental nature of illness, caregiving, dying, and grief is *personal*—and only partly medical. Obviously, seriously ill and dying people have medical needs, but that does not mean that these times in life are fully medical. Yet the health care system responds as if they are only medical. This results in bringing the wrong tools to the job. The personal experience is something that is not antithetical to good medicine by any means. Once you make that distinction, things become clearer and people's needs become easier to meet. Just by naming things clearly, the ability to support them during these inherently difficult times becomes easier.

I would say that training in palliative care has to include experiential training in being fully present—mindfulness training or some other type of centring and self-awareness exercise. It is said so often that it's become a cliché, but it is true: it is not just what you do, it is *how you are*—the quality of being that you bring to the clinical encounter—that matters to patients. That is real. That ability to be fully present and not recoil. To know enough about yourself to know when feelings are your own, rather than them coming from the patient or family. All of that is important.

I see compassion as innate; it can be cultivated, if not taught exactly. It takes some practice. We need to stop teaching it *out* of people. Compassion is a motivating factor that brings the majority of people to health care as a profession. And I think compassion remains the driving force within us. Sometimes the practice of medicine is dehumanizing. The way that medicine is constructed is problem-based so we deconstruct people into their problems and we only see the problems. We need a mixture of approaches but with a focus on experiential. This is what Rachel Naomi Remen from Commonweal calls attention to and what is taught in 'on doctoring' courses in a handful of medical schools (http://www.rachelremen.com). As a doctor, you have to have a certain degree of self-knowledge and self-awareness to do that. Jon Kabat-Zinn's mindfulness practice allows you to have a certain facility with attention that in turn allows you to be fully present, aware of the other person's issues, separating them from your own. And it allows you to keep your heart open. It is so easy to recoil from the pain when you are feeling compassion, that it takes some practice to feel safe and grounded enough to be able to keep your heart open—for instance, to the pain and worry that a mother is feeling in knowing she is going to die and leave her three children with a good-for-nothing father. How do you keep your heart open and be with her through that?

A case exemplar

In all honesty, the case comes to mind is categorically common in my experience. It's a case in which the patient and I became friends in a very authentic way and it was often hard to be with her, because to the extent that I could see her world, it hurt. I accepted that hurt as part of my relationship with her. It is worth it to breathe through the pain and stay present because of that sense of connection. With my patients, I have made this firm decision that I am not going to close my heart—that I will take the pain and I will be with them. I am of a certain age that I know I am going to survive this. I have done this before. I get through it; it hurts but it also feeds me because of the relationship with the other is so rich and that connection, for reasons that I can't claim to understand, is something inherently valuable, meaningful, important, and authentic. That is my compensation in so many ways.

Karen was 14 when I met her, and she died at 17 from one of the more severe cases of cystic fibrosis. With Karen, service to her meant setting my own needs aside, setting a lot of my feelings aside, and showing up even when it hurt, even when she was being mean to me. There was a long time when she did not want to talk to me at all. It was off-putting and testing and that was OK, because it was not about me. So I kept showing up until I wore her down—maybe I proved that I could take it. If there were tangible, pragmatic things that I could do, I would. Occasionally, I brought her flavoured water because she was diabetic due to her cystic fibrosis. She could not have sweet things, but she liked these flavoured waters that they sold in the hospital. I would do that for her as a treat, just to brighten her day a little bit. I am big into 'trinket therapy'. I think pampering people in little ways is really nice, especially when they are in hospital. As I came to know her, I was able to imagine what this adolescent's hard life was like. Together with her, we thought about things that might be of value for her to do. I occasionally got her out of the hospital for an hour or two on weekends, when she was in hospital for weeks at a time. We would go to pet shops because she was so into animals and then have a tuna sandwich or something. Her hero was Jeff Corwin who had a programme on the Animal channel. She just loved this show and him, and it just so happened he lived not too far from us at Dartmouth. One day I said 'Karen, have you ever thought of writing him, maybe you could talk to him, maybe you could see him.' She said, 'He would never answer. . . . How would I get a letter to him?' I said, 'You write it, I will get it to him.' I had no idea. by the way. how I was going to do that but I have done harder things in my life!

It became a project with her and her mom and I helped a bit. I went through his publisher and got it into his hands. By golly, if he didn't respond. She actually went down and spent a day with him in his farm in western Massachusetts. When she came back she hugged me for the first time and she said, 'This was the best day of my life.' This girl did not have a lot of good days. She had a tough life, not only because of her illness. I really believe you could not have got to that therapeutic outcome through the medical model. You had to keep your heart open, remember to breathe and use compassion in the sense of imagination to think about what is possible. I truly believe we are just here to serve. It is not about us, it is about them. We are just here to serve.

Fostering sustainable compassion

I think this has different answers depending on whether the question is political or related to system design. Personally, I would start a citizen consumer movement

and teach patients and families about compassion and give them the tools to recognize it, complain about it when it is not there, be prepared to move their business
and vote with their dollars to reward those health systems and providers that provide compassionate care. Again, I don't think this is about hospice or palliative
care, I think this is about care in general. I am old enough and working long
enough in this discipline to have been blessed to know the founders of the movement, Dame Cicely Saunders, Robert Twycross, Balfour Mount, and others. In the
US we talk about 'wagging the dog'. Early on, leaders in the hospice and palliative
care had a sense that if we were successful we could help transform all of health
care through the example we set. I think we still have that opportunity.

At the same time as hospice and palliative care has matured into the status quo,
we have become the new bureaucracy. Max Weber, the German sociologist, described how social movements that succeeded became routinized with bureaucracy. That certainly describes what has happened with hospice care in the
United States, and it is not a good thing. A new level of creative disruption is
needed. To me, that has to come from the citizen consumers. Nothing peeves the
baby boomers in my country more than thinking they are not getting the best. So
far their expectations are too low. They need to get that sense that well-being is
possible through the end of life. Sadly, they are not. I think the quality of hospice
care in the US has become highly variable. Some of it is still very good; some of it
less reliably so. Most hospice care is given at home through a sequential model in
practice with a reimbursement stream, through Medicare which requires you to
give up disease treatments in exchange for hospice care for you and your family
at home. A large proportion of patients come to hospice late—or not at all.

Today in America, many people are getting bad care through the end-of-life
experience—whether it be hospice care, home care, long-term care, or in
hospitals—and they don't even know it! That is why I say it is not about us—it is
about the people we serve and they are getting short shrift so often for so long.
I try to address this issue in my most recent book, *The Best Care Possible*. It is a
story-driven book that strives to explain the issues and tensions facing people
in America as we strive to give the best care possible to people through the end
of life. I hope it succeeds at least in conveying the feel of the palliative care practice as we experience it today. I want to give those people a sense of what *is* possible and give them the tools to demand it.

Commentary

In the first part of his book, *The Best Care Possible,* Ira Byock makes the important point that 'when someone is seriously ill, a good doctor is a mighty thing'
(2012, p. 28). The attention and commitment to the practice of palliative care

shown through the case presentation of Karen demonstrates just what a 'good doctor' can do to improve quality of life. One of the core messages presented here is that good palliative care practice is derived from a place of service. This may be an uncomfortable concept to embrace professionally, particularly if the sense of service is equated with subservience. However, the idea that we serve others through our careful stewardship of people in need is not new. In a series of essays on the topic of servant leadership, Robert K. Greenleaf (1904–1990) postulates that 'caring for persons, the more able for the less able serving each other, is the rock upon which a good society is built' (Greenleaf 1972: 1). He argues that a better, loving society is only possible if those charged with societal responsibility increase their capacity to serve others. Critical of the failure of institutions, including health, to accept the importance of service, the consequences of rejecting this ideal are complex, uncaring, power-motivated, impersonal organizations that fail to give the best care possible. Sadly, 40 years later, Ira Byock makes the same call for a more 'care-full' society to serve those in greatest need; although both authors reflect their vision of American society, the realities presented are eminently global. Added to this is a system that continually calls for choice but often fails to understand the risks that consumers perceive in having to make certain choices for themselves and the barriers that inhibit engagement—often fiscal barriers, but sometimes based on gender and class (Wilson et al. 2014).

Service speaks not only to compassion but to the idea of well-being in the context of living one's life to the full. The *Journal of Happiness Studies* focuses on academic scholarship in relation to well-being and quality of life. One issue (vol. 9, no. 1), referenced by Paul Gilbert (2010), speaks to the concept of 'eudaimonic psychological well-being'. In this, well-being is demonstrated by being able to reach life goals for the simple pleasure of doing so, rather than because of any perceived reward such as money or prestige. For Gilbert (2010), compassion assists in the development of eudaimonic well-being because it is linked to particular ways of being, some modulated at a neuronal level, others at a more social level, which help to create our self-identity. The kindness and service demonstrated here through the actions of one 'good doctor' help to cement that argument. One US-based organization, Contagious Compassion (http://www.contagiouscompassion.org) also strives to reach that goal. Contagious Compassion is based on the fundamental beliefs that through service, self-awareness and compassion are nurtured and developed, and that student-focused support programmes help individuals to define their personal pathway to service in community. Hopefully, the outcome of such initiatives will start to address the transformation which both Robert Greenleaf and Ira Byock seek: to make living and dying well a caring and compassionately managed experience for them.

Reflections for practice

- What does the idea of service mean to you?
- How do you see well-being promoted within the current delivery of health care and palliative care in particular?
- What are the opportunities available to professionals to foster well-being?
- What are the consequences for the patient and family of not doing so?
- What are the consequences for the discipline of palliative care?

Further reading

Byock I (1997) Dying well: the prospect for growth at the end of life. New York: Riverhead.

Byock I (2004) The four things that matter most: 10th Anniversary edition A book about living. New York, Atria Books.

Byock I (2012) The best care possible: a physician's quest to transform care through the end of life. New York: Avery.

Gilbert P (2010) The compassionate mind. London: Constable.

Greenleaf RK (1972) The institution as servant. Cambridge, MA: Center for Applied Studies.

Halifax J (2014) G.R.A.C.E. for nurses: cultivating compassion in nurse/patient interactions. Journal of Nursing Education and Practice, 4(1), 121–128.

Wilson F, Ingleton C, Gott M, Gardner C (2014) How do perceptions of risk shape 'choice' in end-of-life care. BMJ Supportive Palliative Care, 4, Suppl 1, A20.

Chapter 5

Augusto Caraceni—Roots

Dr Augusto Caraceni is director of the Palliative Care of Pain and Rehabilitation Department and Virgilio Floriani Hospice at the National Cancer Institute of Milan. After graduating from medical school at the Università degli Studi di Milano in1985, he qualified in neurology and clinical neurophysiology at the Università di Pavia. In 1986, while training with Vittorio Ventafridda in pain therapy and palliative care at the National Cancer Institute of Milan, Dr Caraceni participated in the World Health Organisation programme to test and disseminate the WHO ladder for cancer pain relief. In 1994, he was clinical fellow in neurology and palliative care at Memorial Sloan Kettering Cancer Center, New York. Augusto Caraceni served on the board of directors of the Italian Association of Palliative Care and as vice president of the European Association of Palliative Care. His clinical and research experience includes the neurological complications of cancer, cancer pain and opioid analgesics, neuropathic pain in cancer, pain assessment, and measurement and symptom control in advanced cancer, with a special interest in delirium. He has published many articles in indexed journals and other scientific publications, and books in both Italian and English, including a co-authored textbook, *Delirium: Acute Confusional States in Palliative Medicine* (Oxford University Press, 2011).

Foundations in palliative and end-of-life care

I trained as both a neurophysiologist and a neurologist. In Italy we have the opportunity to study clinical neurophysiology at university. While I was doing this, I started to attend the pain therapy unit at the National Cancer Institute of Milan where Professor Vittorio Ventafridda was based. So from about 1986, while studying neurophysiology and neurology, I was mainly involved clinically with cancer pain. After graduation, I kept working in this environment. When Vittorio and others decided to change from a pain therapy and rehabilitation unit to one which included palliative care, I was here and had the opportunity to be one of the staff members. So that is how I started in this clinical area. One significant palliative care experience I had at that time was the development of the World Health Organisation cancer pain relief ladder and the dissemination campaign about getting better treatment for pain for the benefit of advanced cancer patients. I think my transition from neurological medicine was quite natural. That expertise was helpful in addressing pain and from the beginning, Vittorio was already very aware of the needs of patients with advanced cancer being wider than only pain and symptom control. I believe my neurological background was helpful in understanding the full potential of palliative care as a medical practice.

The compassionate practitioner

I considered the definition of compassion by Henri Nouwen and I partially agree with it. It is a very high-level definition, reflective of a higher philosophical description of compassion. It seems allied to a sort of missionary attitude towards the alleviation of suffering. I think it attends to the dark side of our human life. Compassion from a medical and health care professional perspective is something more to do with trying to understand things from the point of view of the patient. As I prepared for this interview, I remembered a section from Cicely Saunders's book *Watch with Me* called 'Not Only Skill but Compassion Also'. The phrase I recall is 'We have to learn how to feel (with) patients without feeling (like) them if we are to give the kind of listening and steady support that they need to find their own way through' (p. 3). I think this is a very cogent definition in which there are two main issues to consider regarding the concept of compassion. The first is about our specific professional perspective. Compassion should be evident in all our actions towards the patient but without invading their personal boundaries excessively and inappropriately. The second is that a compassionate approach should always seek the therapeutic goal evidenced by the expression 'to find their own way through' (p. 3). This rather reflects the ideals of Carl Rogers's concept of unconditional positive regard, where we show complete acceptance and support of the person no matter what. So for me, the compassionate practitioner needs to blend and balance their professionally constructed perspective with personal beliefs and attitudes arising from very profound human feelings, reflecting the whole area of emotion and of being personally close to the patient. How you manage this is complex.

I think there are elements of compassion that can be taught through professional attitudes but it is very difficult where personal attitudes are involved, and these may not be possible to teach. You have to give your focus to the subjective experience of the patient. You cannot demonstrate compassion if you do not take into account the subjectivity grounded in the history, the personal characteristics, and the emotions of each individual patient. I think that you can lead somebody on a pathway which values those aspects of the personality that enhance the ability to understand, communicate and share feelings, particularly feelings that are related to disease, to death, to suffering, and so on. You can teach this theoretically. However, role modelling is a very powerful way of teaching about compassion through practice. By working with experienced people I think you will certainly get the sense of what is really important for patients. Although you can learn from your teacher or mentor, you will probably develop your own way of compassionate practice because of your own experience and ability to learn from patients. In the end, the real learning about how to be compassionate is when you deal with the real individual situations, the real communication with each patient.

I know for others, the presence of a personal faith does impact their understanding and interpretation of being a compassionate practitioner. I have a religious faith, but I don't think that it is instrumental to my practice. I am very aware that my faith is certainly much less strong and more open to doubt and to questions than others I know. Yet—and I think Cicely Saunders is the best example of this—faith was a major driver in leading this very holistic pathway of medicine and health care. In her work, I found that she believed that by helping people through their terminal phase, it would help them to meet God—to see and meet God in real terms. This is the real religious fundament of her palliative care approach. I believe that some of the leaders, and also many of the professionals who work in palliative care, see that faith, religious faith, is certainly a useful, important driver. However, I would have to say that it is not true to say that religious faith is an absolute necessity. I see very many professionals without any faith or religious belief, who practice with a very significant degree of compassion and have the ability to share the very fundamental elements of care with the patient, even having very different beliefs. Faith is not sufficient to make a good palliative care professional or indeed a compassionate one. But the most amazing thing we must remember is that the strength of this faith led to an incredible theoretical and practical approach which we call palliative care but can think of more simply as a compassionate way to address care for patients and families at end of life. That, I think, is interesting.

A case exemplar

I think it is evident that compassion is a constant thread in the way we deal with patients. Not only in palliative care, of course, but perhaps you might expect it to be more visible in palliative care. Compassion warrants a consistent approach. I do not think we should categorize cases as easy, or difficult, or exceptional because there is no limit to suffering.

I remember one case which certainly says something about the challenges of compassion. We had a patient admitted to the hospice; a young man 22 years old. He had been ill since the age of five or six because of an undiagnosed neurological disease but which led to a profound, progressive motor and cognitive deterioration. It was difficult to interpret what type of self-awareness this young man had of the environment, of physical and non-physical sensations and stimulations. His family, father and mother and one older sister, had been living a life totally dominated by the need to care for this young man since childhood. This was particularly the case for his father. He quit his job, so his only occupation was caring for this boy and witnessing the progressive loss of his son's ability to communicate, to talk, to be able to react in any meaningful way or react to any action or external or internal stimulation.

This boy was in a near-vegetative state, although he could still be fed by mouth. He had significant difficulties, which only the parents seemed equipped to overcome. It was very difficult to understand how they managed. Then, after all this, he was found to have untreatable metastatic cancer. Some early treatment was offered but then it was decided that it was not possible to treat the cancer anymore and that it was appropriate to have him admitted to the hospital for palliative care. He had a large thoracic mass invading one of the lungs so we expected difficulty in breathing. Pain was also a probable concern but that was very difficult to interpret because of his neurological disease.

The whole therapeutic planning was very, very complex and difficult because whatever we did or suggested, the parents were always blocking us and intervening in his care. It was all very intrusive, particularly his father who was constantly checking things. To give you an idea, if he was running a fever, he would measure the temperature every 20 minutes. The father kept a diary. He was filming his son's reactions to show us that this young man was showing some conscious appreciation of what was going on. Our clinical evaluation was that it was almost impossible to assess and interpret the needs of this young man. We wanted to provide some pain relief based on the assumption he might have pain; we wanted to help with the complexity of his symptoms; we wanted to let this family understand that he was dying. This was so difficult for the staff and for everybody in the hospice. The paediatricians were trying to keep a link with them but the family was very angry and aggressive with them because they thought that it was the paediatricians' fault that the diagnosis was made late and he could have been saved.

We had to cautiously negotiate any treatment, any minimal interventions that we felt were important for the patient, trying to interpret his vocalizations so that he was not suffering. The parents didn't want us to give medications and we were afraid that by not doing so, we were leaving him to suffer. This left me with a dichotomy: how can you bear that suffering as a parent? How can you bear the suffering as a professional? How can you know what is the right course of action when you don't understand very well what is happening to the patient and there are different interpretations of it? I think you reach such a level of, in a sense, powerlessness, impotence, and total weakness professionally and personally. When every potential effective action is taken away from you, you are left with a total lack of ability to respond, whether as a doctor, a nurse, or even from a personal point of view. You reach a point—I call it the 'final land' where you have to release the tension in some way, you and the patient and family.

I think that is where compassion comes to the fore. It helps to ground you when the situation is extreme and you find yourself unable to intervene. The extreme complexity of that situation may let the intuitive response, which is compassion, emerge. You have to strip away so much to get to that point, where all the different people and feelings can meet. The best you can do is agree to try to do the best you can, and I think we were able at least to do something. We feared that when this young man died, the father was probably going to go crazy. I think that he dealt much better than we thought, and afterwards he came back to thank us. Now we have lost track of him, but I do believe that something meaningful happened for us all.

I think this experience brings me back to the definition I quoted earlier from Cicely Saunders, which is this idea of feeling with people without feeling like them. That was the compassionate response needed here. I think there is an inevitable sharing of the suffering of other people. When patients and relatives suffer in your presence, you have to look at its impact on you at the same time and therefore you can experience the negative feelings of suffering and loss. As a health care professional, you have to consider the meaning and impact of this suffering with your professional lens. I think, again, this is very much demonstrated in Cicely Saunders's experience when she describes the profound feelings she had with some of her patients and family experiences. You experience the loss but have the ability to go back, to develop a creative way of dealing with it in a professional manner. But it will never prevent you from experiencing subsequent loss. Loss is always present.

I think a significant challenge for us in this case was the lack of resources available for debriefing or supervision. We discussed it at a weekly meeting on Tuesday mornings, but unfortunately only the people on duty participate in the meeting. I think that we had the opportunity to meet with our psychologist who was helping with some of the counselling in the hospice, but that was only on occasion. The staff schedule doesn't allow for this type of specific time to be allocated. We tried to address what happened, as we did in other cases. But a systematic way of managing this is just not available to us at the moment.

Fostering sustainable compassion

I am the director of the Department of Palliative Care of Pain and Rehabilitation and the hospice part of a very large cancer treatment centre. This poses both challenges and opportunities. Some of the challenges are very practical because we are constantly competing for resources, trying to educate the other doctors and nurses to improve their communication with patients, to improve their ability to facilitate the transition for patients from the active phase of treatment to the palliative phase of treatment with limited resources. Globally, I think everyone here experiences the challenge of dealing with incurable cancer. If we compare ourselves to 20 years ago, there is far better recognition of the benefit of palliative care and that is a significant change. At least there is nobody saying that palliative care does not help at all or does not even exist. I think an important opportunity has been the independence, recognition, and respect that the palliative care service has gained in this institute over very many years. I do think that whatever model of specialist palliative care you develop, it is about having a level playing field to be able to have a dialogue with the rest of medicine, with the other specialities, because dialogue is based on two people. You cannot talk to yourself. The ability to have that dialogue face-to-face is what is important. I think we have a very specific role in challenging where the patients are not informed realistically about their prognosis or cannot find somebody who is able to talk about end-of-life issues with them. To sustain compassion, I think mutual dialogue enhances opportunities for the rest of medicine to have real physical contact with palliative care. It opens the opportunity to develop a shared language around that part of care, which can be forgotten by modern medicine. Unfortunately, this is not always valued in the process of building modern medicine because resources are not allocated to that. Medicine is evaluated for its scientific publication and clinical throughput of patients, not necessarily its ability to care.

One question to be considered, of course, is whether there is now a distance between the original message of hospice as proposed by Cicely Saunders and what may be considered a more professional approach to palliative care as a part of more mainstream health care beyond her original inspiration. Any development where there has initially been a strong vision can diminish the revolutionary zeal or originality of the message. But I think that there is much more benefit to this than burden.

The original inspiration of Cicely Saunders was the engine to start a change in professional health care practice—to make these elements active into what it is now the professional delivery of palliative care. The fact that in a cancer institute like ours we have a full section dedicated to palliative care shows that we have the opportunity to work in such a way that palliative care can moderate the technological excesses visible in modern medicine. It can help the system look at *this* side of medicine, which accepts that death, by its very nature, will always be. I have seen many ways in which palliative care has been made real in health care systems and yet stay true and consistent to the original ideal. Cicely Saunders herself was a champion of introducing palliative care into health care systems. Although she said that she would very much like to help patients to meet God, she also stated that she would be satisfied if she could improve the level of care of the dying in the health care system. So for me, there is no tension between her vision and aspirations and the desire for palliative care to be integrated into mainstream care delivery. She has said this message in so many ways: her vision that hospice is made for care, education, and research; her contribution the *Oxford Textbook of Palliative Medicine* where she made this very call. She was profoundly rooted in something that has to do with an alternative conception about the science of medicine and technology not being apart from the patient's subjective experience, from the patient's profound feelings. Perhaps somebody whose professional interest is in cancer biology mechanisms, hoping to solve the problem of cancer as a disease process, may be less interested in what people think and feel. If you implement palliative care into any health care system, your starting point is probably different. And so is the impact that you are going to have. We have found that when both junior and experienced doctors and nurses in oncology have the opportunity to be with us, to see the compassionate delivery of palliative care, many find something that is relevant for their practice, for their personal way of being a doctor or a nurse in whatever field they work.

This brings me back to where I began this discussion. Much of my discussion is reflected in Saunders's small booklet *Watch with Me: Inspiration for a Life in Hospice Care*. The quotation at the beginning of this chapter arises from a conversation that she had with a patient in the last days or weeks of life: 'I look for someone to look as if they are trying to understand me'(Saunders 2003: 3). This woman wants people to know she is dying and that she is accepting of that fact. What is important is Cicely's subsequent comment that this is not about sentimentality or sensationalism: this is about the reality of living and dying. For me, compassion is also not about sentimentality or sensationalism. It is something that is both relevant and important to our everyday practice.

Commentary

As a neurologist, Augusto Caraceni would find the current interest in the neuroscience of compassion a valuable discourse. The e-book by Singer and

Bolz (2013), *Compassion: Bridging Practice and Science*, provides not only a contemporary discussion about compassion in its broadest terms, but also an overview of the research which is looking at the scientific basis of compassion at the level of brain and endocrine and immune system function. For example, studies have noted the positive effects of compassion meditation on distress responses. Researchers are also investigating the neuronal correlates of compassion; notably, what happens in the brain when one gains new perspective regarding self and others. The endocrinology and immune-system response of compassion are also developing fields of study.

Like many of the contributors to this book, Augusto Caraceni makes reference to the roots of palliative care arising from the work of Cicely Saunders and how that vision transformed the delivery of care not only in Italy but across the world. He points to an important understanding that sustainability of compassionate palliative and end-of-life care is based in its potential for development and growth. He argues that the presence of a palliative care service in proximity to other disciplines is important in being able to guide the complex transitions between living and dying. He also notes in the clinical case, the challenge of feeling powerless when care is rejected and the need for the team to have some outlet to explore that in a constructive professional way. Concern that the interface of palliative care and mainstream practice has in some way diminished the original message of hospice is not borne out here. Rather, Cicely Saunders herself advocated that the vision of hospice care was for all in need of pain and symptom management, including those in hospital. The A.B.I.D.E. model of compassion (Halifax 2012) proposes an adaptive system in which to see the interrelational, mutual, and reciprocal nature of compassionate engagement. Such engagement fosters the dialogue, which Dr Caraceni sees is necessary for compassion to be a part of everybody's professional work.

Reflections for practice

◆ Do you believe that the original message of hospice care is as true today as in its original inception?

◆ What are the questions that you would need to ask in order to evoke a compassionate response to the family situation in this clinical case?

◆ What are the questions you would need to ask yourself?

◆ What do you consider to be the added value of palliative care to the wider health care setting?

Further reading

Caraceni A, Grassi L (2011) Delirium: Acute confusional states in palliative medicine. Oxford, Oxford University Press.

Halifax J (2012) A heuristic model of enactive compassion. Current Opinion in Supportive and Palliative Care, **6**(2), 228–235.

Rogers C (1951) Client-centered therapy: its current practice, implications and theory. London: Constable.

Rogers CR, Stevens B, Gendlin ET, Shlien JM, Van Dusen W (1967) Person to person: the problem of being human: a new trend in psychology. Lafayette, CA: Real People Press.

Saunders C (2003) Watch with me: inspiration for a life in hospice care. London: Mortal Press.

Singer T, Bolz M (eds.) (2013) Compassion: bridging practice and science. Munich, Germany: Max Planck Society.

Chapter 6

Carlos Centeno—Lessons learnt

Professor Carlos Centeno works as a consultant in palliative medicine at the University of Navarra Clinic, with special interest in clinical research topics such as fatigue and symptom evaluation. Since 2002, he has led a European working group that studies the national development of palliative care across the European Union, and with the European Association for Palliative Care has published the Atlas Palliative Care in Europe and, more recently, a similar atlas for South America.

Dr Centeno currently directs a new research programme called ATLANTES at the Institute for Culture and Society, University of Navarra, which applies the approaches of humanities and social sciences to advanced diseases and palliative care. Dr Centeno also teaches postgraduate courses in palliative medicine at the University of Navarra and other universities. He has authored a *Manual of Palliative Medicine* for students and has published numerous papers in international peer-reviewed scientific journals.

Foundations in palliative and end-of-life care

I am 51-year-old physician, working full-time in palliative medicine for the last 17 years. I completed my residency in radiation oncology but I always thought about working in palliative medicine. I think I went through oncology looking for palliative care. Oncology offered a great preparation because at that time, the terminally ill patient was cared for mostly in oncology. From the very beginning, I knew I would always be a palliative care physician. My decision to work in palliative was based on my conviction that palliative care is the right way to approach end-of-life care. At that time, in 1992, palliative medicine was only beginning in Spain. There was very limited work in the field and yet, clinically, it was a real necessity. Today, it is still a necessity but there are hundreds of teams in Spain working in palliative medicine. So, for me, the decision to work in palliative care arose from a personal conviction that it is necessary to teach others about this way of caring. After medical school and before any clinical work, I completed my doctoral studies and the topic of my PhD was the psychosocial needs of the palliative patient. My understanding of the patient from that research led me to work in palliative care as a health care professional. I decided to dedicate my professional life to the development of palliative care in my country and internationally. Now my time is spent mainly in clinical work. I see patients every day and I also teach in the university. I am in charge of the palliative medicine programme in the bachelor of medicine degree in the University of Navarra. For the last two years, I have been leading a programme of research called ATLANTES within the Institute of Culture and Society in our university. It is about social science and humanities in palliative care. The project has two main foci. The first is about the foundations of palliative care; the second is to develop strategic projects to improve the understanding and perception of society towards palliative and end-of-life care, and has an international focus regarding the practice of palliative care around the globe.

The compassionate practitioner

For me, to be compassionate in my work as a palliative care physician is to have the capacity to be able to be with the patient in his or her suffering, to be by their side, as a person, not just a physician. Not just a doctor in a white coat but that ability to be a human being present to people's suffering. I believe that the greatest support a patient can receive is the presence of another person wanting to help him in spite of the suffering. That means having the capacity to match your inner self with that of the patient so that the patient receives the support he needs. By being present to your suffering, I can help you. That is my idea of compassion.

I read the Henri Nouwen definition to my team this morning and the physicians and nurses understood what I was talking about. They understand compassion in English as being able to be moved by the suffering of another person. However, in Spanish the word *compasión* has a rather negative connotation. It has this sense of pity for a person, more than, say, the idea of an unlucky situation or when people say, 'What a pity'. If you are talking about compassion as that the strong internal feeling in response to the suffering of others, then the Henri Nouwen definition is broad enough and probably valid but not very concrete in its description.

I believe my compassion comes not from faith but from my personality, my personal way of being. Faith is helpful for me to feel compassion. It perhaps augments compassion, but this compassion is not just from my faith. Compassion reinforces my faith and through compassion, I can try to be more like Jesus Christ in the way that he was with people as the perfect human being: through compassion I can look more like him. Compassion comes from within. Perhaps I see compassion in my life in this way because many times I feel from my faith that I am an instrument. I don't know if that makes sense to you. I am the instrument, not the instigator of things, something is happening through me. And sometimes I experience that the love of God is coming through me. It is a kind of symbiosis between faith and personality, I think. By being a good Christian I am a better doctor and being better as a doctor, I think I am also a better Christian.

The way that I explain compassion to my students and clinical fellows who visit my unit are that we all have an internal 'elastic membrane' that vibrates and moves, responding empathically to the suffering of the patient. With time and experience in palliative care, you find this membrane becomes increasingly flexible. And so you become more perceptive to the suffering of the others. Some people ask me, 'How can you work every day in that area?' And I explain because this membrane is flexible and moves me deeper and deeper towards the suffering of the patient, when I stop for a moment to evaluate and I think positive thoughts such as 'I think I've really done all that I could to help this patient' or 'That is very beautiful' or 'Thank you, God, for this experience', the elastic membrane recovers to its original position. And then you are able to work with the next patient because you are ready for this kind of experience again. That image sustains me in my practice. When I see one of my students in conversation with the patient, perhaps tearful, I tell them, 'Don't be worried about this, this makes you a better doctor.' Only when you experience that level of deep emotion can you truly help the patient. I really think my greatest strength as a physician is the capacity to perceive suffering and to try to be in resonance with the suffering of the other.

I used to believe that compassion could only be taught through presence and experience. Bedside teaching was the only way to show compassion and I certainly use that method. I teach compassion to my students through reflective discussion after we visit the patient. In that way, the students perceive what I, the professional, experience and feel. They see how I am moved by a particular situation and how this medical professor not only teaches me about the disease of the patient but he also demonstrates the human elements of practice, talking about the feelings and the support of the patient. In that way, I think that the students can fully understand compassion. More recently, I have taken this a step further, getting them to reflect more deeply on the situation after observation. So, after observing an interaction in the room of the patient and the small debriefing that we have outside the door on leaving, I ask each member of the team to reflect on two questions: what they see and what they feel, and to give me one word to describe what they have observed and felt in the room. And people share that they feel uncomfortable, they feel at peace, they feel good about themselves, etc. The students go deeper into the concept of compassionate caring for a patient. So, this mentoring is one way to impart compassion.

The second approach I use to teach compassion to the student is through the use of a DVD. I have a DVD of a patient, a young woman, who wanted to talk about her disease to help others in the future. It was very powerful. It was like a window opened in her heart. It is a wonderful record. And I use the same DVD for all my students every year. After the DVD, I get the students to reflect and discuss what is happening in the room. This is a two-hour workshop and many students tell me they find this very helpful to them. Real-life films of patients can teach compassion because if a patient can share their deep feelings, the student begins to understand that this is the normal way of being to help others. Of course, the third way to teach compassion is through the formal course curriculum. One of the nurses on my team reminded me of that when this morning we were preparing this talk. To have palliative care as a topic in the curriculum gives you the opportunity to demonstrate the importance of personhood and this perception correlates well with what I receive from the students in the written reflection at the end of the course. They tell me exactly the same, 'Through this course, I have learnt about compassion.' I don't know if that is true but they have certainly seen it in practice.

A case exemplar

I can tell you of one case where I think compassion is present in the current work I do. The patient was a woman around 60 years old. She had spent many years of her life in spiritual work overseas, promoting a religious institution in that country. She presented with a relatively slow-growing brain tumour but eventually she and the family decided not to go further with chemotherapy because she was very depressed. The tumour had left her unable to speak and although she seemed to lack some awareness, she was very able to understand. I met the patient at Christmas because the family were very concerned about their ability to care for her and so they called me and I decided on an immediate admission. I monitored her for several days but quickly realized that the patient was more or less the same way she had been on her last visit several weeks previously and that the clinical situation was stable.

After one week, I proposed that the family should consider transferring the patient to what you call hospice, but which here in Spain usually means a residential care centre or nursing home for the elderly. The family agreed and I made my last visit to the patient before the transfer to the nursing home. For many days, when I spoke with the patient, I would tell her not to be worried that she was unable to speak because I could read what she needed to say in her eyes. I needed to reassure her that I understood what she was experiencing. I believe that the patient understood what I was trying to tell her. I tried to convey that sense of being with her by reinforcing that I could sense her needs from the way she looked at me.

And then the patient smiled, tried to say something. I remembered that this person was a very religious person and so I explained to the family that, three or four days previously, I had the experience that when the patient started to cry, her expression told me that she was moving all her spiritual resources to try to accept the suffering. I had a strong sense that something had changed for her emotionally. I explained this experience to the relatives in her presence to encourage them to pray with her because I felt that prayer could be one way they could support her to do things that might be important to her, such as being able to converse with God. When I said this, the patient started to cry again and I could see her trying to move from that place of pain to where she felt more in control. And then I saw her smile again. The doctor who was visiting the patient with me for the first time told me that she found it a beautiful visit.

A lovely ending to this story that I wanted to share was that chaplain told me shortly afterwards that when he gave her the sacrament of anointing, she began to sing a popular song, because although the tumour prevented her from speaking, she could still sing and the chaplain knew that. So, I suggested that the relatives should not speak too much or pray normal prayers, but perhaps it would be more helpful to read a section of the Gospel or play a song and sit in silence with music playing. Then, after the music stopped and some time in silence, read the Gospel and then put the music on again. I knew that this patient had spent a part of every day of her life in meditation and this helped her to meditate, just in a different way.

Fostering sustainable compassion

Because I am a palliative care consultant in a large oncology centre, every one of my patients is under the care of the oncology team and many receive chemotherapy. I also see palliative care patients in the oncology day hospital where patients receive oncology treatment and palliative care at the same time. I don't think that it is a question of the kind of treatment that the patient is receiving that denotes whether care is compassionate or not. Perhaps when you are alone with the patient and it is clear that little more can be achieved through active oncology treatment, it is easier perhaps to talk about different topics. I suppose sometimes expectations that something positive may come from the chemotherapy or the oncology treatment is unrealistic. There can be limitations or challenges when the patient or family do not want to talk about palliative care or is too unwell or too close to death to engage with you fully. Sometimes the patient does not speak Spanish so they cannot discuss these deeper issues with you. I suppose oncology treatments can be a limitation in the way compassionate palliative care can be offered but, for me, compassion is mandatory, it is not an option. It is the only way to care for the whole person. You as the practitioner have to be compassionate whether people are receiving chemotherapy or not.

We should consider this in light of our palliative care roots. We have to do many things in palliative medicine today. Research is extremely important. But we must not lose the fundamental vision of the pioneers in the world, such as Cicely Saunders. One of my projects is to keep the history of palliative care alive because it is a powerful way to show all health care professionals the fundamental foundations of palliative care. There is a book about the history of palliative care in the United Kingdom by David Clark and colleagues (2005). That was wonderful idea to me and so I hope to do a similar project in Spain with my colleague, Javier Rocafort. Through studying the life of the pioneers, you can see the diversity of backgrounds, some of them religious, some not, but clearly spiritual people doing very visible compassionate care. Through the life of the pioneers you can perceive the foundations of palliative care. And so, my proposal to sustain compassion is to keep the personal history of the pioneers alive, especially Cicely Saunders. A couple of years ago, we translated her book *Watch with Me* into Spanish. From the moment I translated this book with my friend Enrique Benito, I realized as a Spanish doctor that the life of Cicely Saunders is an inspiration to us. I realized what powerful words Cicely Saunders gave us to instil within us the capacity to be compassionate with the patient. Through that translation, I feel greater compassion towards my patients and I think it could perhaps be helpful for other physicians to reflect, to read, and understand the practice of Cicely Saunders.

I think that in order to sustain compassion, we need to be more reflective about the language of compassion. We need to be able to express it more clearly; the differences between compassion as emotion and compassion as action. There is a really valuable article by Harvey Chochinov (2007) published in the *British Medical Journal* where he explains that compassion may arise from a number of sources, including the personality, personal experience, or training. If compassion can have several sources in your life, you can always grow in compassion from several sources. So, taking time to get a better understanding of your personal sources of compassion may help you to find your own inner compassion and apply that in practice. That would be really valuable.

Commentary

In an important article by Harvey Chochinov (2007) on the idea of dignity conserving care, he cites the experience of the writer and literary critic, Anatole

Broyard, at that time living with metastatic prostate cancer. Broyard wrote, 'To the typical physician, my illness is a routine incident in his rounds while for me, it's the crisis of my life' (Broyard 1992: 43).

Chochinov argued that a person's dignity, their self-perception of value and worth, is intimately related to the way in which health care professionals affirm that worth through looking beyond the illness to the person who is now labelled as a patient. The ABCD mnemonic (attitude, behaviour, compassion, dialogue) draws its reference from the writing of Francis Weld Peabody, a Harvard-based physician who, in an address given in 1927, wrote that 'the secret of the care of the patient is in caring for the patient' (Peabody 1927). The reflections of Carlos Centeno echo much that Chochinov writes about compassion in this model. It speaks to an understanding of one's own vulnerability in the face of another's suffering. It develops over time and with clinical exposure so that the intuitive response (e.g. the sense of being able to see what the patient without speech wishes to convey) becomes the stepping-stone to a deeper engagement with the clinical experience. It is, above all, an acknowledgement of our frailty in the face of the clinical ambiguity that often challenges us in the care of people at the end of their lives. Carlos Centeno offers an inspiring discussion on how compassion can be imparted through mentorship and teaching, using a breadth of resources. The advent of educational technologies in clinical teaching will no doubt enhance such resources for the future. What is vital to embrace compassion more fully is exposure to the world of medical humanities, the arts, and social sciences to truly understand the illness journey of the patient. Chochinov argues this as essential to understanding what dignity truly means. To do that, we need to understand how compassion and dignity interplay in the expression of our clinical practice and the extent to which this reflects my essential humanity as opposed to any professional role that I may hold. Reading the words of those who live the experience of dying may be the most important lesson learnt.

Reflections for practice

- Take time to write and reflect in some detail on a clinical case where you feel that a patient's dignity was not upheld. To what extent could that have been avoided by utilizing a compassionate response to the situation?

- Consider the case using the ABCD model. How do the elements of attitude, behaviour, and dialogue reflect the ideals of compassionate care?

Further reading

Broyard A (1992) The patient examines the doctor. In Intoxicated by my illness and other writings on life and death. New York: Ballantine.

Chochinov H (2007) Dignity and the essence of medicine: the A, B, C, and D of dignity conserving care. British Medical Journal, **335**, 184–187.

Clark D, Small N, Wright M, Winslow M, Hughes N (2005) 'A little bit of heaven for the few?' An oral history of the modern hospice movement in the United Kingdom. Lancaster: Observatory Publications.

Peabody FW (1927) The care of the patient. Journal of the American Medical Association, **88**, 876–882.

Picardie R, Seaton M, Picardie J (1997) Before I say goodbye: recollections and observations for one woman's final year. New York: Henry Holt & Company.

Chapter 7

Mark Cobb—Suffering

Mark Cobb grew up in Manchester and after studying for an engineering degree at Lancaster University worked on a development project in Swaziland. He returned to the UK to study for ministry in the Church of England at Ripon College Cuddesdon, Oxford, and trained in the diocese of London where he began to specialize in health care chaplaincy working at the Marie Curie Hospice and the Royal Free Hospital. From there he furthered his training and experience in acute health care and palliative care at the Derbyshire Royal Infirmary and Macmillan Palliative Care Unit. He moved to Sheffield as head of the Chaplaincy department at the Royal Hallamshire Hospital and is now a clinical director at Sheffield Teaching Hospitals NHS Foundation Trust where he heads a directorate of over 400 allied health professionals.

Mark's education across science and the humanities enables him to span disciplinary boundaries and engage with different fields of enquiry. His primary academic interests are in palliative care, for which he was awarded a PhD from the University of Liverpool; his research portfolio includes spirituality, health service design, and medical ethics. He holds honorary academic appointments at the University of Sheffield and the University of Liverpool, teaches undergraduate and postgraduate courses, and has a wide range of published works notably in the area of spirituality.

Foundations in palliative and end-of-life care

I have been working in palliative care for about 22 years. After training for ministry in the Anglican Church, I served my curacy in London and part of that work was to support a fairly large hospice. I had no particular drive or interest in the field but it came as part of my duties, so I would go to the hospice for a number of sessions a week. I had the support of a very senior chaplain who ran the team in the hospital. To be honest, it was a case of 'now you are here, this is part of your duties; get on with it.' I soon realized that it was an area that held a lot of interest for me. It really kind of grabbed hold of me and was an area of my work that I wanted to understand in much more depth; it was an area I felt I could make a difference in. In this particular hospice, I was instantly expected to be a member of the team and could have been asked to go and sit with someone who was dying and alone. I witnessed how my colleagues in the multidisciplinary team coped with this work and how they processed their reflections. The team were generous enough to share that with me and to help me to think through the issues and questions which arose. My supervisor was an experienced hospital chaplain, well versed in supervision, and he would let me bring cases to work through. That really helped me.

After I finished my curacy, I wanted to go into health care chaplaincy and to develop my practice in palliative care. At the time there were a couple of joint posts between general acute hospitals and hospice/palliative care units. It meant I then had proper time to develop my practice and to further my learning and training within the palliative care world. I was able to access all the training that other clinicians could obtain as well as pursuing more specialist training as a chaplain. For example, St Christopher's Hospice used to run the hospice chaplain course which included sitting at the feet of Cicely Saunders herself and listening to her pearls of wisdom. She used to do one-to-one sessions with you as well. You came across a lot of people who were part of that initial pioneering movement, trying to get people to understand what a hospice was. Broadly speaking, the vocational drive of individuals who opted into this movement was very tangible. These were very driven people with a real passion for palliative care. Palliative care was still fairly new, so people were still feeling their way, trying to consider what a palliative care unit was and how it operated. There were not many models to go with except St Christopher's Hospice in London and Cicely had her experiences in hospitals and with religious communities that ran infirmaries. Really, St Christopher's was modelled on a small hospital—not quite that scale, but in terms of the environment and layout. So in that sense it was quite helpful to be around those people. These were formative influences with highly regarded practitioners, and in this case the founder of the whole movement, as well as powerful experiences with patients.

I suppose from a chaplain's perspective, ministry around death and dying is not particularly pioneering—it is what we do. I did not have to argue for my role or what I would be doing because that is what chaplains did. As the hospice movement developed and more units began to appear, chaplaincy into hospices became much more professionalized and organized. These days, whilst I am sure parishes and other faith communities continue to support hospices, most UK hospices or palliative care units will appoint and employ their own chaplain or chaplaincy team. These appointments will take account of the demographics of the population the unit is serving and typically be informed by the professional guidance of the Association of Hospice and Palliative Care Chaplains. Chaplains normally need to be licensed to practice or have the approval of their faith community. But the appointment is made by the hospice who would select, appoint, and employ the best candidate.

The compassionate practitioner

For me, to be compassionate is to have a capacity for a truthful encounter with people who are facing the end of life. We often talk about compassion in relation to suffering, and I think that is true, but I think it is also about people who are concluding their lives. There is something very important for me about the final phases of life however we define that, because it does vary. For some people, it is an incredibly focused period of their lives. People will sometimes describe it as a holy moment, a holy place. Coupled with that is the more traditional definition of compassion as the emotional and ethical response towards the person. It is not just about witnessing it but it is the response given to that—that is what compassion is. For me, from a Christian point of view, it is about a faith response, derived from the belief that God is not dispassionate and remote. As a Christian, I would say we know God through Jesus who came to be with us and who responds to us. As we seek to follow in that pattern there is a vocational sense of calling to be compassionate and that is a demand of faith. I can completely appreciate that people can be compassionate without having any faith at all and to do so from an emotional and ethical point of view. I derive part of my capacity for compassion from my faith because I feel able to do this work as it does not just stop with me. I hand it up to God.

I believe nearly all people have some innate capacity for compassion but if people have damaging experience they can self-protect and without support it can be quenched. It has to be nurtured and fostered in the right way, particularly when you are younger in your career; it has to be done in a way that is safe. We have all seen people who have been brutalized through their training, and they never recover and function primarily in that self-protection mode. I realize I work in a self-selected group but I do believe we have a sensitivity and openness built into us—that ability to imagine what the suffering of others is like and to imagine what one is going through.

It seems to me that the strong Christian background of Cicely Saunders has become something of an embarrassment and almost been whitewashed, partly because people do not know what to do with it. It is very clear when you read her selected writings; it is absolutely fundamental to her vocation to establish hospices and underpins everything that she believed. We have somehow got to a position where all that has become boxed away and disconnected from where we are now. Perhaps through the process of everything becoming formalized and professionalized, the original *charism*, to use a real theological word, has served its purpose and fades. We need to rediscover the *charism* again. I think Cicely Saunders used quite strong theological language which we would find difficult to use these days. The whole subject is now framed by the language of spiritual care within health care literature. We no longer talk about the Christian roots of caring in the hospice movement but we now talk about spiritual care, existential issues, and issues of belief. It is interesting that most of the time it is clinicians and health professionals who are having these discussions. Maybe it is that we have to keep rediscovering and finding new language to do so. Part of this plays into the whole societal shift, where people have become dissociated from religious institutions and therefore are no longer familiar with the language. Yet the fundamental human issues that all religions deal with are as relevant as ever—such as the meaning of death.

I don't think you can teach compassion. I am drawing purely from my own experience in observing and witnessing other people who are wise, reflective practitioners, recognizing their capacity for compassion and their responses to people who are suffering and being able to learn from them and reflect with them. I think to understand compassion needs experiential learning, the kind of novice-to-expert apprenticeship. It is learned by being with and learning from others. It can be hard to ask for help and support so you could provide some sort of structure which enables people to work alongside experienced practitioners, building in theories of reflection, perhaps exercises to help develop their compassionate capacity. In some sense I think you should formalize things. Many of us had to fend for ourselves and managed to hopefully come out on the right side of that. That is where putting together some kind of programme is helpful. In training people in chaplaincy, we sometimes use the phrase 'to foster people's pastoral imagination'. This is the ability to understand another's situation from a pastoral point of view. This resonates with the whole movement of humanities in health care, getting people to open up to other people's worlds and perspectives. The inclusion of a humanity subsidiary to an academic programme would have a lot to offer, through literature, theatre, and the arts. In chaplaincy, we generally offer placements for chaplains who are training but have experimented with placements for other professions such as clinical nurse specialists and registrars. I suspect the people who come with me have been self-selecting and been able to leave aside their own professional perspectives to learn what a chaplain's perspective is in palliative care. We have had some very enriching discussions after we have been to see patients around that.

A case exemplar

This was a man in his early 40s, married with two children, late primary school age, so old enough to understand what was happening but young. He was admitted to the hospice with advanced disease and was expected to die within a week. He had a lot of unmanaged symptoms so he was in a lot of physical distress and his family were equally distraught. At the time of admission, it felt like the number one objective was crisis management. When he first came in, a very strong case was made at the multidisciplinary team meeting for therapeutic sedation until he died. The physician in charge wanted to try to get some of the symptoms under control to see if they could stabilize him a little more. On admission he had made clear that he and his wife were practising Christians, and wanted to see a chaplain. He was referred to me as an urgent case, framed by this clinical background of someone who was dying and a family in need of support. I thought my brief was clear—to prepare for his death. What I was faced with was a family in a crisis of faith, feeling that God had let them down. For them, this was not part of their life plan. They had followed the tenets of their faith and this was not part of it. I was challenged to respond to their question of how God can let people suffer and die in this situation. It is a fairly standard for a chaplain to be involved in a situation where people have a faith that has worked for them until they hit a crisis and then it falls apart. They have never needed to think about it because they have never been in that situation before. They often don't have the internal resources to deal with it.

One of the things he kept asking of me was to listen to him talk about his faith. It is not that usual for someone just to want you there to listen. I could not work out what this was all about at the time. Fortunately, the team were able to relieve a lot of the distressing physical effects of his disease. His wife could not deal with the distress and she found it very difficult to be in the room with him. It was not easy to watch what was going on. Thankfully as the symptoms were managed better, she was able to spend more time with him. This brought the emotional tension down and began to open up some space for him again.

This was a man who knew the Bible backwards which was a challenge for someone like me who does not come from that tradition. I think initially he felt unable to let go of the story that had kept his family going for many years. His wanting to tell me his story was an outlet to show he was still capable of reaching out beyond this immediate physical insult to another person.

Part of his gift to me in sharing his faith story and understanding of the Bible meant that the space which opened up between us allowed me to share some of how I understood the Christian story. We were able to discuss passages in the Bible around suffering and get him to see those in a different way. This enabled him to move away from this rather mechanistic view that 'I have been good so God should be good to me' and we really focused around the story of Jesus and what happened to Jesus. God's son suffered but was held in all of this by God and by God's love. That began to bring the resolution.

Suffering can really collapse a person. It can really oppress them. They just don't have any space to be who they are. When people are in distress it is very hard to think of anything else. Part of the work of the chaplain is to hold situations to try to open up space where people can feel comfortable and confident to explore situations and issues. Through that, we were able to further explore the story of Jesus. Rather than abandon the view he had before, he was able to see it within this bigger horizon of God holding suffering; suffering is part of God's world; it is not alien to God. Therefore he was able to have the confidence that God was still there. Whereas when he came in he felt abandoned by God, and as God's representative, I was held to account for that.

This case really alerted me to this issue of capacity. I don't think I fully understood that at the time. It is about needing to give people those spaces, to still be who they are and not just look at this very distressed, physically symptomatic individual who is losing most of who they are as a person. This case also challenged me to expand my understanding of compassion. I think I had come to this case on one emotional level—I could sense the distress in the room, so I felt I could respond from a place of compassion in that sense. What this case called me to do was more than just that—it was saying this person needs an encounter with another person, beyond the emotional distress and suffering. It was that person wanting someone else to hear his story, to acknowledge the truth of who he was. To be authentic and to have those encounters of truth is very demanding.

Obviously, chaplains are trained in liturgy. The tradition this family came from was very ritualistic and so one of the things I was able to do as a chaplain was to hold a Eucharist in the room and we broke bread. As we moved to a place where he and his family could see suffering as part of God's will, which God holds and responds to in love, the Eucharist seemed a natural next step because it expressed that liturgically through ritual. The fraction of bread is a highly symbolic and theological act which speaks about the brokenness of Christ and which for this man and his family's faith tradition was highly resonant. It was an incredibly powerful moment in an episode of end-of-life care. We held the Eucharist the day before he died (not that we knew that at the time) and his family spoke about the blessing and gift it was for them all. With people of faith, the Eucharist is always a profound sharing, both in terms of human solidarity, the communion with ourselves but also with God. At the centre of it all is this brokenness; we share the wholeness of God through the breaking of bread. Good liturgy can speak much more than words can.

Fostering sustainable compassion

The longer you spend in the company of people who are dying, the more you are confronted with your own mortality. Part of maintaining your compassion is to be comfortable living in a body that is mortal. It is one of the gifts I found of working with dying people; they have taught me how to do that. Of course, we encounter people who don't accept that and struggle with it to the end. You also meet people who have reconciled themselves to their mortality. That is something I have had to learn.

For chaplains, the things you rely upon such as your prayer life and spiritual discipline are very important for your well-being and being an effective part of the team. It is very easy to leave that to one side and just focus on what is in front of you when demands are high. Unless you are replenishing, you get burnt out. In palliative care, we are blessed that team work is seen as so vital; discussing a patient as a team is very helpful in giving people the opportunity to unburden in a safe way. As members of a team who go through similar things, it is safer to share because you know others will understand where you are coming from.

I have heard the debate played out amongst nurses that we have lost the soul of nursing—we have become medical technicians. There is a real attractiveness to people in health care about shiny, technical things. For me, it is always going to be about the humanity of care, and I wonder, with the current shift in society, how the next generation will see one another—what kind of exposure will they have to issues about suffering. I am very mindful to the fact that there is a lot of suffering portrayed in the media but it is always very remote. Cicely Saunders was of a generation where people fought and died in wars or suffered from diseases now eradicated.

So, for me, an important question is what shapes the present generation's view of suffering and human interaction? I would say we risk losing compassion, but in the sense of working in incredibly strained services. I think people do the best they can with the resources they have available. It is not that they are deliberately uncompassionate, or that they have forgotten how to be compassionate. We have not changed the conditions in which hospice care is delivered, but hospices today often use the same language as acute care. There are always patients waiting to come into a hospice and so the pressure is to admit, control symptoms, set up a good management plan, and discharge back to the community or nursing home as quickly as possible. There is a possible shift in focus and hence you get people talking about the patient flow, the lack of time. I am not saying that everybody should die in a hospice but I do think palliative and hospice care has become much more technical because there is so much more available. Much of this is of real benefit to patients but we must never let that distract us from that humanity of care. This needs time and attention and it is hard for me to see how you can attend to that at the same time as managing complex technical demands. It is important to give time to people who have little time left.

I do think the arts and humanities foster people's imagination. I guess part of the future is how to engage people empathically in the reality of suffering. If you look around the world, we can be overwhelmed by the scale and extent of suffering. You need to bring it down to a much more human level. I used to interview applicants for medical school, who now have to demonstrate some experience of caregiving such as working in a care home. It is really quite revealing for some of them and opens up space for self-reflection. They start to feel for caring rather than it being just a technical thing. Their compassion is fuelled by that kind of emotional acknowledgement. When you are young it is quite hard to sense that but I know we try to select people who have a natural desire to care rather than just be academically capable of completing the course.

In the Christian theological condition, the whole issue of the existence of suffering and the goodness of God comes under the heading of theodicy. Some of the most important work around suffering and evil was done following the Second World War. Prior to his execution in Nazi Germany, the German theologian Dietrich Bonhoeffer wrote letters from prison reflecting on these kinds of issues (Bethge 1997). He was very instrumental in beginning to shift some of the Christian theological position on suffering and God. I suspect Cicely Saunders was aware of this kind of theological discussion and was trying to work that out herself. I think that comes through in some of her writings.

Compassion is the realization of our responsibility for our fellow humans. I teach chaplains that you will be exposed to a lot of suffering and you have not only to understand that at a human emotional level but also theologically. Suffering is challenging personally and theologically; it can be hard to reconcile beliefs with experience, and I have seen new chaplains who have not been able to reconcile that and left for other types of ministry. The capacity for compassion takes years. You constantly have to work at it.

Commentary

To try to understand compassion leads inevitably to our understanding of, and response to, suffering. However, the relationship between compassion and suffering is complex and has been the subject of much philosophical debate. Amongst those arguments is the extent to which those faced with another's suffering suffer themselves (Nilsson 2011). As Mark Cobb shares in this chapter, suffering is oppressive and debilitating. It is also in the nature of our shared humanity that we are open to alleviate the oppression and debilitation of suffering in our fellow human beings. John Donne (1572–1631) expressed that connection in his work 'Devotions upon Emergent Occasions', where he says, 'Any mans death diminishes me, because I am involved in Mankinde' (Meditation 17, 'No man is an Island'; http://www.gutenberg.org).

In an address on East-West monasticism shortly before his death, the Trappist monk and philosopher, Thomas Merton, concluded, 'The whole idea of compassion is based on a keen awareness of the interdependence of all these living beings, which are all part of one another, and all involved in one another' (2002: 45). Therefore, as proposed by His Holiness, the Dalai Lama, this interconnectedness means we hold a collective responsibility to care for others and 'promote the happiness and peace of all beings' (2011: 7).

Looking at the case exemplar shared, those involved in the delivery of palliative and end-of-life care are involved at some of the most intimate and challenging moments of suffering in human life. In practice, they face the dilemma and struggle associated with the realization of human mortality. In *Living Buddha, Living Christ*, Thich Nhat Hanh notes that 'looking deeply together is the main task of a community or church' (1995: 77). Mark Cobb shares how, in listening to, sharing, and honouring stories of differing traditions, the ability to heal and bring peace in the midst of suffering is eminently possible. This is not about what I (the practitioner) can do for you (the patient). Rather it is what we can do together by the simple virtue of our same-ness that can respond to the pain of suffering in a compassionate way.

This chapter also provides a clear exposition on the contribution of chaplaincy to hospice and palliative care work. It offers deeper understanding around the spiritual dimension and clarifies how the specific skills and attributes of chaplaincy serve the patient, family, and team. As health care professionals, there is learning in considering what the presence of someone who has a specific role in spiritual care evokes in us, both positively and negatively, and how we respond to that.

The ability to develop and lead meaningful ritual which comforts, guides, and strengthens those who suffer is an essential part of managing life's ending (Myers 2003). Thomas Moore defines ritual as 'an act that is performed primarily for its symbolic and imaginistic import and for its effect on the soul' (1996: 157). There is evidence that ritual is important in people's lives and we, as health care practitioners, have a responsibility to ensure that this is respected and facilitated wherever possible. It may also form an important part of self-care for professionals working with dying patients on a regular basis as a way to acknowledge the impact of loss and grief on the caregiver (Running et al. 2008). The ritual of shared Eucharist expressed in this case and the representation of the brokenness of Christ echoes the description of compassion offered by Henri Nouwen as entering into broken places of others' suffering. It is important to see that sharing—that sense of 'fraction' as Mark calls it—can lead to a blessing and gift in terms of healing and understanding.

Reflections for practice

- ◆ How important is having a faith or personal belief system for you in the practice of palliative and end-of-life care? If important, how does that sustain you? If not, what ways do you sustain yourself in the clinical care setting?

- ◆ What does ritual mean to you and how could that be expressed in the practice of palliative and end-of-life care?

- ◆ How do you see the role of the chaplain or spiritual adviser in your team? How is that honoured and respected in your clinical service?

Further reading

Bethge E (1997) Dietrich Bonhoeffer: letters and papers from prison. New York: Touchstone.

Hanh TN (1995) Living Buddha, living Christ. New York: Riverhead.

Dalai Lama (2011) How to be compassionate: a handbook for creating inner peace and a happier world. London: Atria.

Merton T (2002) Love and living (NB Stone, Br. P Hart, eds) Boston: Houghton Mifflin Harcourt.

Moore T (1996) The re-enchantment of everyday life. New York: HarperCollins.

Moore T (2002) No man is an island. San Diego: Mariner.

Myers GE (2003) Restoration or transformation? choosing ritual strategies for end-of-life care. Mortality, 8(4), 372–387.

Nilsson P (2011) On the suffering of compassion. Philosophia, 39, 125–144.

Running A, Woodward Tolle L, Girard D (2008) Ritual: the final expression of care. International Journal of Nursing Practice, 14, 303–307.

Chapter 8

David Currow—Courage

Professor David Currow initially trained as a physician in internal medicine and undertook sub-specialization in palliative medicine. At the same time, he completed a Master of Public Health. He was the foundation chief executive officer of Cancer Australia, the Australian government's national cancer control agency. He now leads the New South Wales government's agenda in improving coordination of cancer control through improved service delivery models, reduction in risk of cancer through lifestyle change, evidence-based population screening, and targeted research investment. He continues as professor of Palliative and Supportive Services at Flinders University, Adelaide. He is the principal investigator on the Australian government–funded Palliative Care Clinical Studies Collaborative, the world's largest clinical trials group in palliative care. Previous roles include national presidencies of two peak bodies, Palliative Care Australia and the Clinical Oncological Society of Australia.

With more than 300 publications to his name, David Currow was recently rated one of the top ten most published palliative care researchers in the world. His impact is evident in policy and service development, research, and teaching throughout Australia and internationally. He is a senior associate editor of the *Journal of Palliative Medicine* and an associate editor of *Bio-Med Central Palliative Care*.

Foundations in palliative and end-of-life care

Essentially, I came to work in palliative care by accident. In 1990, I was assigned as a senior resident in my third year after qualifying to a term of palliative medicine. In palliative care, there was no registrar. I absolutely loved it. I did it for three months and decided to do another three months just to make sure I convinced that this was what I wanted to do. From that point I went back and completed my internal medicine training, and then subsequently specialized in palliative medicine. I have been involved in palliative medicine in one way or another for more than 20 years. So, to be honest, I stumbled across it and fell in love with palliative medicine. I would still say the same today. My work in palliative and supportive care at the moment is entirely research-based. I am a principal investigator on the National Palliative Care Clinical Studies Collaborative;

a series of phase 2, 3, and 4 clinical trials. I am the co-principal investigator of CareSearch (http://www.caresearch.com.au) which is the evidence-based website that the discipline runs from Flinders. It gets more than 30,000 visits a month. I am also the co-principal investigator at the Palliative Care Outcomes Collaborative, the national quality improvement initiative that explores variations in clinical care from point-of-care data collection. It is a benchmarking/feedback loop to drive improvement in clinical care.

The compassionate practitioner

I think compassion is a very difficult thing to define. There is an element of empathy, being alongside people, and projecting oneself into their situation, really trying to understand how you would want to be supported were you in that situation. It's trying to understand things in that person's situation from their point of view, from the suffering that they are experiencing in the context of their life rather than bringing one's own life views to that interaction.

I think that compassion is a human trait and health professionals have generally come to their role with a sense of helping others, reaching out to people, wherever those people are in their life journey. We need to ask if there is there something particularly *different* about palliative care from the rest of clinical care. If it is a universal human trait, then what is it in palliative care clinicians that is amplified? Personally, I think there is a real challenge saying that palliative care has something special. Many of my colleagues outside of palliative care practice with immense compassion under very difficult circumstances, and they are not looking after people at the end of life. I think particularly of those in psycho-geriatrics, drug and alcohol rehabilitation, the emergency room—particularly those doing emergency surgery—those people are extraordinary. They approach their practice with a compassion that I admire and hope that I can bring to my clinical encounters. So, I have to say I don't think there is something special in palliative care, because I see it in other disciplines just as often. We are all part of the human spectrum. We have days where we are probably not as compassionate, not as 'present'. If you want to be compassionate you have to be present, in that broad sense of presence; really tuned into that person. We all have times where we have not quite made it there, for whatever reason. On other days, we hope we do it incredibly well.

People connect in different ways, and as a result of that have different conversations. There are clearly some people with whom we can relate that other members of our teams may not and vice versa. In exploring compassion, we have to rely on team-based care and not beat ourselves up if we are not as connected to each patient as we perceive everyone else on the team to be. If I am really honest, I think one of the biggest challenges in palliative care is that we don't trust our team colleagues to have those conversations. For truly compassionate care, we must trust that patients will have those conversations with the right team member, at the right time, and that may well not be with every team member. Not every person can have the same presence, the same co-suffering, the same empathy with every single patient. If we set ourselves up with that belief, we will fail ourselves and our patients.

That said, we know that better communication skills can be taught and there is good evidence that you can improve communication skills: the process of listening, processing, and responding.

If we accept that compassion requires presence, then ultimately presence is about listening to the subtext and cues. Inasmuch as we can improve those skills, we can also improve the ability for someone to acknowledge that there may need to be a compassionate response. I can't teach someone about suffering, as such, but I can do a great deal to improve junior clinicians' ability to pick up the cues of suffering: the unspoken, the body language, the intonation, the uncertain questions. We can improve our compassionate radar, as it were—the antenna we tune to do this.

I think the flip side of that is also true, and that is that compassion alone is not sufficient to be a good palliative care clinician.

There is a great quote by C.S. Lewis. 'I had been far more anxious to avoid suffering than to achieve delight!' (Lewis 1955: 220). If you consider the quotation on compassion by Henri Nouwen, those emotions and attributes are all in the downside of things. I think one of the things we miss in palliative care is that being alongside someone present is also celebrating the good things, being excited by the things that have made this person happy today, helping them celebrate the reconnection with someone in their life. The definitions we use for compassion are so built around suffering, we must not forget that there are many happy and joyous moments in palliative care, as there are in the rest of life. I don't think that we in hospice/palliative care are as comfortable, sometimes, in getting alongside people when they are happy and celebrating.

I think there are people who came to palliative care believing that all you had to do was have compassion. The evidence suggests that patients want clinicians who are technically competent as well. If you look at the list from Karen Steinhauser's research on what is important at end of life, first patients want physical symptom control, in order that they can do all these other things (Steinhauser et al. 2000). I think there are people in hospice and palliative care who honestly believe you do not need those broad range of skills because compassion in and of itself should be enough. This is not the case anywhere else in clinical practice—in any discipline. Being compassionate is not sufficient. Compassion can only have its full effect if we bring to bear everything else we know that can improve care and outcomes for this person. It is no mistake that the WHO chose to define palliative care twice and to include concepts like 'impeccable assessment' (World Health Organisation 2002). That is a very, very deliberate set of wording, particularly in the most recent definition. So yes, we need compassion, as any health practitioner needs compassion, but we need technical competence, as any other practitioner needs technical competence.

A case exemplar

In this case, I may have been influenced through reading some Scott Peck, very popular in the 1990s. I think it was *Further Along the Road Less Travelled*. I think it is an important book because of the parallels between psychosexual development and psycho-spiritual development. It's fascinating and it has helped me immeasurably at the bedside. There was a women in her 60s and I had seen her a couple of times in clinic. She was an inpatient and we just could not get on top of her symptoms. She was not sleeping, pain was a problem, fatigue, nausea, constipation—you name it. Nothing I did seemed to be making any difference at all. There was a ward round. I sat down with her. I did not even put a question; I put an open statement, 'You look scared.'

I just stopped. I didn't say anything else and I just let the silence sit with it. Over the course of the next 20 minutes she started to talk to me. She talked about the fact that she was afraid, and we started to talk about those fears. Finally, I took courage in my hands and I said, 'Let me go out on a limb here and you can stop me at any time, but just let me ask you something,' and I said to her, 'You are really angry with God, aren't you?' I don't talk about God with patients. I can if I have to, but it is not something I do. She looked at me and she said, 'Yes, how did you know?' I said, 'You are cross with God because he only does good things to good people and bad things to bad people.' Her face changed. I said, 'You can't talk to anyone about this either, can you?' She said, 'I can't talk to my pastor about this, that would be a lack of faith. I am angry with God but I am not allowed to be angry with God because he is going to punish me for being angry with him.' That was the crux of the conversation. We talked on for another 20 minutes. We had a fantastic pastoral care worker at the time. She came and spent time with her every day.

Some extraordinary things happened, but I think part of compassion is the courage to be there. You need to think why you would try a question like that, in that circumstance. There were cues, but there was nothing specific. I think a message from Henri Nouwen's book *The Wounded Healer* was that issue of courage. I don't think you can have compassion without courage. The courage occasionally to do something totally different in order to try to be alongside that person in a way you normally are not. Being out of one's comfort zone is not a passive and pleasant process. It is not hand-holding. It is having the real desire to be in that person's shoes in order to try to help them in a way that another health professional, family, or in this case the clergyman, was going to be unable to do—because of barriers she had put up, because of beliefs she had—perhaps because of the beliefs and barriers her clergyman had put up.

Fostering sustainable compassion

I wrote a reflective piece a few years ago with a nurse colleague, Meg Hegarty where we argued that we use so much of our empathy and compassion with our patients, we run out of it with each other as palliative care clinicians. We have some of the most uncompassionate, un-empathetic people in this field when dealing with colleagues. I moved states a few years ago and when I arrived in the new place, people said to me, 'Palliative care is a circular firing squad.' We have so much compassion for our patients, but not when it comes to each other. I actually think we are pretty good at compassion with our patients. I think we are pretty good at supporting their families. I think we are really good at supporting our colleagues outside palliative care. I am just not sure if we have enough compassion for some of our colleagues inside palliative care. I think people who have not done some time in oncology are likely to be far more critical of oncologists who are giving third-line therapy. My response to that is, 'Have you sat over from the other side of the desk to someone who says I have responded so well to second-line therapy when you told me it wasn't going to work? Have you actually had that conversation?' I don't think we have enough compassion for our colleagues within palliative care and I think we have some particular targets outside palliative care towards whom we are not terribly compassionate either.

I have heard the concerns of over-medicalization. I have written on that and prefer the term over-professionalization. It is not just medicine. Not everyone who is dying needs to see a specialist palliative care service. I have argued that at a policy level the idea that you can't die well without seeing a palliative care service is the ultimate demonstration of over-professionalization. We published a paper in *Palliative Medicine* on referral to palliative care in 2004. We identified four groups of people: those who need it and get it, those who don't need it and don't get it, those who need it and don't get it, and those who don't need it but get it.

We have got to be really honest about that and get the hell out of trying to see everyone because we believe we are so superior to all of our colleagues. Again, it's the view that we, and we alone, can provide good care in this setting. A lot of my colleagues struggle with that because if we are not seeing them, who is?

I think this debate is an incredibly important part of our discourse and we must watch that very carefully. In the end we all need to bring our very best skills to supporting people at this complex time of life. At the same time, we do not want to create problems—we do not want to light fires in order to put them out.

Sometimes I think we focus on wanting to hear everyone's life story. That may or may not be part of good care in that circumstance. That is why compassion is so important. We have to understand from this person's point of view, their problems and concerns, and not try to impose our views and our needs.

For the future, I think we need to take compassion as a component of clinical palliative care but not an end it itself. Earlier, I spoke about teaching compassion through better communication skills. I think the other area where we can own our compassion is by working at our self-awareness. We have a lifelong role in refining our self-knowledge, our reactions, our views, and our responses in order to fully be able to relate to those around us. Things that can help us come alongside people more effectively include reflective practice—creating the time and discipline to do something in a regular and structured way to help address our own personal existential questions. However, I stress not necessarily to share the answers with anyone else, but to know what it feels like to struggle with the questions.

I think in palliative care there has often been the assumption that we should be able to handle anything that comes along because we are palliative care professionals. Actually we should *not* be able to handle everything that comes along. This work is difficult.

I started to introduce this concept into the team I worked with in the late 1990s. At first, there was a fair bit of resistance; then four of the clinical nurse specialists and one of the nurse consultants started to have regular debriefing as a group once a fortnight, apart from the other people on the team. The change that I saw over the next 12–18 months was amazing, in terms of team and people's practice. It was absolutely fantastic to watch.

I have seen the same person for supervision since 1997. This person challenges me and does not let me get away with stuff. They say, 'David, we have had this conversation, why on earth are we back here again?' Some time ago, I looked after a relatively young mental health professional who was dying of advanced breast cancer. I would walk in and she would say, 'I know the next question you are going to ask.' That is how she started. I needed to think if I could do anything here which may help. I went to a supervision session on Saturday morning and all we did was focus on this particular woman. I did a ward round that afternoon, and I got further in 20 minutes than I did in the previous four months. Supervision works. I really believe that we have a responsibility to get this right in the context of our colleagues who have incredible compassion in providing the same beautiful diligent care that so many health professionals came into the profession to provide.

Commentary

Cameron et al. (2013) investigated the ways in which physicians communicate compassion to their patients. From this small-scale qualitative observation study, they developed a taxonomy of behaviours associated with compassionate medical practice: recognizing suffering in the other person; creating an emotional resonance, often through the use of silence; and moving towards addressing that suffering if at all possible. David Currow echoes those findings through the clinical cases presented here. The ability to listen attentively and meaningfully to what is said and unsaid is a skill which underpins the daily practice of palliative and end-of-life care. Robin Youngson contends that such compassionate listening 'radiates a powerful field that reassures, comforts and calms others' (Youngson 2012: 113). A powerful lesson for practice given by David is that courage is an essential element of the compassionate response of the health care professional. He refers to this specifically in this chapter. Diasaku Ikeda, founder of Soka Gakkai International, a Nichiren Buddhist lay organization, considers that compassion without courage is not genuine. They are inextricably linked and cannot be separated. In palliative care, knowing when to act or not can be an equally courageous step. Those decisions are made based on the wisdom of clinical experience. Perhaps also they come from what the Torah describes as 'qol dmanah dagah,' which can be translated as a whisper, a soft, murmuring sound, or, in the Book of Kings (19: 6), 'the still small voice'. Rabbi Michael Comins calls it 'the voice of fragile silence' (Comins 2001). Developing the sense of knowing intuitively the right course of action to take in a given situation is an essential part of palliative care practice. Believing that takes courage.

Reflections for practice

◆ What do you think it takes to be a compassionate and courageous practitioner? When courage fails, why may that be?

◆ Consider the clinical case of the woman in spiritual distress as discussed by David. How would you respond? What does this case tell you about the compassionate practitioner?

◆ Is there an example in your professional life when your clinical decision-making has been drawn from 'the still small voice'? What is the message from this experience for your practice?

Further reading

Cameron RA, Mazer BL, DeLuca JM, Mohile SG, Epstein RM (2013) In search of compassion: a new taxonomy of compassionate physician behaviours. Health Expectations. doi: 10.1111/hex.12160

Comins M (2001) Elijah and the 'still small voice': a desert reading. CCAR Journal: A Reform Jewish Quarterly, 47(2). http://www.torahtext.org

Currow DC, Abernethy AP, Fazekas BS (2004) Specialist palliative care needs of whole populations: a feasibility study using a novel approach. Palliative Medicine, 18, 239–247.

Heschel AJ (1955) God in search of man. New York: Torchbooks.

Ikeda D (2004) Unlocking the mysteries of birth and death . . . and everything in between: a Buddhist view of life. Santa Monica, CA: Middleway.

Lewis CS (1955) Surprised by joy: the shape of my early life. Orlando, FL: Harcourt.

Mishneh Torah [English] http://www.chabad.org

Nouwen H (1979) The wounded healer: Ministry in contemporary society. Colorado, Image Books

Peck Scott M (1998) Further along the road less travelled: The unending journey towards spiritual growth. New York, Touchstone.

Steinhauser KE, Christakis NA, Clipp EC, McNeilly M, McINtyre L, Tulsky JA (2000) Factors considered important at the end-of-life by patients, family, physicians and other care providers. Journal of the American Medical Association, 284(19), 2476–2482.

World Health Organisation (2002) Palliative care. http://www.who.int/cancer/palliative/definition/en/

Youngson R (2012) Time to care: how to love your patients and your job. Raglan, NZ: Rebelheart.

Chapter 9

Julia Downing—Seeds sown

Professor Julia Downing is an experienced palliative care nurse, educator and researcher, with a PhD that evaluated palliative care training in rural Uganda. She has been working within palliative care for 24 years, with 14 of those working internationally in Uganda, Africa, and Eastern Europe. She is an honorary professor at Makerere University, Kampala, a visiting professor at Edge Hill University, and an international palliative care consultant working with the International Children's Palliative Care Network and as part of an EU-funded project to develop palliative care in Serbia. She has extensive experience in research, presenting at conferences, and writing for publication, and is on the editorial board of the *International Journal of Palliative Nursing* (*IJPN*).

Professor Downing serves on the boards of several international NGOs including the International Association of Hospice and Palliative Care. She is on the Board of Hospice in the Weald and the African Palliative Care Association UK, and is vice chair of the scientific committee of the International Children's Palliative Care Network. She is also an honorary research fellow with the Department of Palliative Care, Policy, and Rehabilitation at King's College London. In 2006 she was the recipient of the *IJPN*'s Development Award.

Foundations in palliative and end-of-life care

I initially trained as a nurse in Cardiff at the University of Wales College of Medicine and I went to work straight away in oncology, trained as a cancer nurse and then in palliative care. I worked across a range of settings in oncology, inpatient, acute, chemotherapy, chemotherapy day unit, haematology, radiotherapy, outpatient, and palliative care. So, quite a broad oncology-haematology background.

Two things brought me into palliative care. Before I qualified, I was working as a student nurse in a medical ward and there was a patient who was dying in the main part of a Nightingale ward and they moved her into one of the side rooms. It was really evident that the staff did not know how to treat this woman. They crept past the room and were not going in. There was this fear of people not knowing what to say and how to cope with this person who was dying. It really struck me then that one of the things I wanted to do as a nurse was to be able to support patients in whatever situation they in. So right from my training there was this seed sown for me about being there for people when they were going through difficult times, being there for people and their relatives as they were dying. As part of my training, I had an elective period at St Christopher's Hospice and there I was able to see the other end of the spectrum to what I had seen earlier on in my training. To see the quality of care that was provided and the difference you could make to the life of patients and their families who were dying, going through that very difficult time. I think those two extremes really helped to sow that seed in me for palliative care. Even though I did not go in to palliative care straight away, that seed developed within me over the coming years. When I qualified, I went and worked in oncology in the UK and then got involved in palliative care and HIV care and eventually went out to Uganda, worked across Africa, and now in Eastern Europe.

My interest in Africa stemmed from another elective in my training when I was talking to a friend at church who was linked to a mission in Africa. So I applied to the mission organization to go and do my elective in a hospital, in a place called Luampa in Zambia. I spent three to four months out in Zambia and fell in love with Africa, but felt I wanted to have more experience to be able to train others and teach if I wanted to go back and work in an African context. I came back to the UK and got experience as a nurse, did my teaching qualification to teach at university level, and so on. There was still this seed sown in me, not just for palliative care, but for Africa. It all came together and I went out to work in an education and clinical training site for HIV and palliative care in Uganda in 2001. I lived in Uganda full-time for ten years and for the last three and a half years I have been part-time in Uganda and part-time in Eastern Europe, specifically Serbia. In Uganda, I am one of the first two professors in palliative care in sub-Saharan Africa, and the only nurse. I work with the Makerere Palliative Care Unit and the palliative care team at Mulago Hospital, providing clinical supervision and work alongside them on the wards. I am also involved in education and service development and work with other palliative care providers including Hospice Africa Uganda (HAU) and the African Palliative Care Association (APCA). I am also involved in research and as I work with the International Children's Palliative Care Network, I am involved in children's palliative care in Uganda, Serbia, and globally.

In Serbia, I am part of an EU project to develop palliative care. The people involved in that heard about the work we had done across Africa and asked me would I consider going to help and share some of the experiences, skills, and knowledge that I had gained in developing palliative care in low-resource settings. I think both cultures are very different, but in trying to develop and set up palliative care there are similarities—limited access to medications and prescribing rights, the need to educate the public and the policy drivers, for example. So, my work is quite varied.

The compassionate practitioner

For me, compassion is probably at the core of palliative care; I think it is the essence of being a palliative care practitioner. For me it is about walking with people, being with them, and not being afraid to be with them. When I was training as a student, I saw that staff were afraid to walk with people going through that palliative care journey. For me it is about being sensitive and not being scared to enter into others' suffering. By walking with them and entering into their suffering then you can show that compassion, you can show that care. I think it is a lot more than clinical care. I think you can be very good at managing pain and symptoms but if you don't do that within a compassionate frame, you can't provide that palliative care. It is that important bit about walking with people through that difficult pathway of being human and understanding that.

I think one of the things about the Nouwen definition of compassion is that it is all quite negative—it talks about pain, brokenness, fear, etc.—but compassion also asks us to go where it is joyful, to go with people through the good times. It is not all about pain and anguish and I think as a palliative care practitioner that is supportive. If it was all about pain, fear, and hurt, then it would be almost impossible. As we show that compassion, we also share in those joys, perhaps when a broken relationship is healed, the good things like that.

For me, compassion comes from my Christian faith which is very important to me. Despite the fact that I consider palliative care has its roots in Christianity, there is not really a lot written about Christianity and palliative care. The way that Christ showed compassion to all those that he walked with and in the way he met people where they were—that is the model for me of how to be a compassionate practitioner.

We talk in palliative care about holistic care and the psychological, social, and spiritual needs of the patient, but when it is about being a compassionate practitioner, it is about us. We have to think about ourselves in that holistic nature and what that means for us, not just the patient. It is easier to show compassion in certain situations than others. Sometimes, it is harder because of conflicting episodes in our own lives. Being a compassionate practitioner has a cost for us as individuals as well as benefits. That is why it is important for me that we see the joyful things in compassion, and not just the painful things. I think being compassionate is about giving part of yourself and not holding back. Giving a bit of yourself will make all the difference for the patients and their families. That can also be hard for us as practitioners. I was trained that you don't get upset when patients die and you only show your professionalism. Being compassionate is about getting that balance between being a professional and being a human. I have always said that the day I don't feel the loss of that person, that human being, that loved one—that's the day I leave palliative care—that is when I will know my compassion is not there anymore.

I think you can develop compassion but I am not sure if it can be taught as such. One thing about compassionate care is that you really need to be able to demonstrate it. It is not really theoretical training, it is more demonstrating through mentorship, through supervision—so by demonstrating compassionate care, by teaching around therapeutic communication, then you can develop and promote compassion. We have a challenge in Serbia because there are not many places where you can take people to demonstrate clinical practice. We have worked alongside colleagues from Romania in the new palliative care unit, working with Serbian staff trying to demonstrate compassionate palliative care. As an example, a Romanian nurse was able to show a Serbian colleague how to engage with a distressed patient and not shut the conversation down for fear of making them more upset. Therapeutic relationship is important in compassionate care. We have been doing quite a lot of communication skills training demonstrating empathy, compassion, and respect through role play; trying to create an environment where they can explore some of these things and try to learn from that.

A case exemplar

There was an African woman referred to us from the National Referral Hospital. She was aged 24, had both AIDS and cancer, and she was dying. She also had fungating wounds which smelt very unpleasant. She was lying on the bed in chronic pain, isolated and alone. One of the impressions people have of Uganda is that everyone has their extended family to look after them and for the most part, they do. However, you come across patients where it is really hard for their family members to cope. Although it is improving, the stigma of AIDS and cancer persists so, for whatever reason, this woman had been abandoned by her family at this stage. We did have access to some morphine and so could manage her pain. But you could see from her face it was more than physical pain. There was this spiritual pain but as she did not speak English, I could not talk to her directly. I had to talk through other people. On this particular day, I spent about half an hour with her and held her hand, I talked to her in English and I am not sure what she understood. I was just able to sit there and be with her. She died about three days later. However, before she died she said the fact that different members of the team, myself and others, spent time with her and just sat there with her made such a difference to her because she felt valued and loved. To me that was an expression of compassion. There was not a lot we could do from a medical point of view, but the fact that members of our team showed compassion at different times made a difference to her. Compassion involves awareness of the need to do something beyond the intention. It is that action. It is not just a feeling.

Fostering sustainable compassion

I think there is probably two parts to that: how do we as health practitioners provide this compassionate care and what we can do to foster compassion among health professionals working both in palliative care and the wider health care system. The health system is all about numbers seen, length of stay, and the focus is on different areas than what we think about in terms of compassion. We have got to look at the systems in which we work and how we can make those systems more amenable to providing compassion. It is not just the number of patients that we have seen but the outcomes of care. We always talk about palliative care as having the patient and the family at the centre, and yet we recently looked at models of care in Malawi, Uganda, and Kenya and did not see patients and family at the centre in many of the models of palliative care that we provide. It was more about the health care professional. So, I think it is about trying to get back to ensuring that the patient and family are at the centre of the care that we provide and how that is visible within our health care system. If you keep the patient and the family at the centre, you will show compassion within the provision of palliative care.

There are specific challenges for resource-poor countries in this regard. In Uganda, I was horrified by the sheer number of patients that needed palliative care, especially the children. I have this vivid memory of a paediatrician from the United States on placement here. I saw him in the morning of his first day and he was really looking forward to it, bright and bubbly. I went down to the canteen at lunch time and he was there with his head in his hands. He said, 'In the last three hours I have seen more children that are dying than I have seen in the past 20 years of my career.' How do you get that balance between the fact that you give of yourself, but have to look after yourself as well? We need to promote an environment where we can support our staff. When I was working in oncology/palliative care in London in the Oncology Unit, they offered staff four complimentary massages from therapists over a six-month period. It meant an hour for ourselves, enabling us to have that time and space and to continue to work in that difficult environment. I think there is part of the system trying to support the staff in different ways; some people have support groups, other people have one-to-one meetings. I know there has been research done on the type of people who work in palliative care and we often tend to self-select the people who are able to cope with that giving of ourselves. Personally, I find palliative care very rewarding because you can make a big difference to the lives of individuals and their families at that difficult time. I think if you just focus on the negative, the suffering of others is going to burn you out. If you think of the positive difference you can make—an individual has died well, in good circumstances, pain-free, etc., with the family there—that sense of satisfaction or reward that you have been part of that process means that giving of yourself can be so rewarding. I find if you tell people you work in children's palliative care, they say, 'How can you work with children when they are dying?' Yet the fun you can have—I know that sounds strange—but you can have fun with the children even when they are dying.

I think for many of us there is often a trigger or something that gets us involved in palliative care, something that ignites the compassion or whatever it is, and at times we need to rekindle that and remember what is it that got us into palliative care in the first place, what sowed the seeds of compassion. It is not always easy, is it? But if we can remember what started us off in that journey, that can help us to continue to grow in our compassion.

Commentary

The idea of 'seeds sown' as expressed by Julia Downing is a metaphor which resonates with the idea that compassion is something deep within us that can be nurtured and encouraged to growth through careful tending. Sakyong Mipham Rinpoche, author and leader of Shambala meditation and retreat centres worldwide, wrote, 'Whatever we do lays as a seed in our deepest consciousness and one day, that seed will grow' (Mipham 2006). All who contributed to this book have shown how those seeds of compassion have grown in themselves and been nurtured by others. Important to that growth is the ability to care for oneself and to embrace the ideal of self-compassion. Self-compassion proposes that the approach to being compassionate to others' suffering equally applies to us. 'Self-compassion is simply compassion directed inward' (Neff & Germer 2013a: 493). Drawing from Buddhist perspectives, Kristin Neff has described self-compassion as comprising three elements: kindness, a sense of common humanity, and mindfulness, the latter of which has grown exponentially in palliative and end-of-life care practice as a way of self-preservation. There is a significant body of new research in the area of self-compassion with the development and validation of self-compassion scales and the impact of programmes such as mindful self-compassion (MSC) and mindfulness-based stress reduction in dealing with mental suffering (Neff & Germer 2013b; Shapiro et al. 2005). A small-scale randomized controlled trial by

Neff and Germer demonstrated that participants in an MSC programme could improve their self-compassion by 43 per cent, or by 1.13 points on a 5-point scale. A clear distinction between self-compassion and self-esteem is drawn, the latter often related to how people compare themselves to others in terms of, for example, success or failure, happiness or sadness, and physical attributes. This can be challenging and destabilizing, resulting in dysfunctional behaviours such as prejudice or narcissism for its maintenance. Self-compassion derives from the sense of equality in being human (perhaps what Henri Nouwen calls 'the condition of being human'—see Introduction) and offers greater emotional stability than self-esteem alone. Julia Downing is not alone in suggesting that being able to see joy amidst the suffering of others is important in our personal capacity to engage in palliative and end-of-life care over an extended career. Being able to see the joy within the encounter between practitioner and patient, even in the context of suffering, may help to start a journey towards self-compassion as the antidote to fatigue and burnout. Sowing those seeds early in a career can lead to an abundant growth in later professional life.

Reflections for practice

◆ Consider the doctor that Julia Downing encounters who is overwhelmed by the number of children dying. How would you foster a compassionate response to this person's sense of futility?

◆ How important is self-esteem in your professional role and what are the benefits and burdens associated with that which may challenge your ability to be a truly compassionate practitioner?

◆ If you were to sow one seed for your future development in palliative care, what would that be?

Further reading

Mipham S (2006) Ruling your world: ancient strategies for modern life. New York: Crown Publishing Group.

Neff K (2011) Self-compassion: the proven power of being kind to yourself. New York: William Morrow.

Neff K, Germer C (2013a) Being kind to yourself: the science of self-compassion In T Singer, M Bolz (eds) Compassion: bridging practice and science. Munich: Max Planck Society. 492–499.

Neff KD, Germer CK (2013b) A pilot study and randomized controlled trial of the mindful self-compassion program. Journal of Clinical Psychology, 69(1), 28–44.

Shapiro SL, Astin JA, Bishop SR, Cordova M (2005) Mindfulness-based stress reduction for health care professionals: results from a randomized trial. International Journal of Stress Management, 12(2), 164–176.

Chapter 10

Betty Ferrell—Empathic entrée

Betty Ferrell, PhD, RN, has been in oncology nursing for 37 years and has focused her clinical expertise and research on pain management, quality of life, and palliative care. A professor and research scientist at City of Hope in Los Angeles, she is a fellow of the American Academy of Nursing and she has over 350 publications in peer-reviewed journals and texts. She is principal investigator of a programme project funded by the National Cancer Institute, 'Palliative Care for Quality of Life and Symptom Concerns in Lung Cancer', and principal investigator of the end-of-life nursing education consortium project. Dr Ferrell is a member of the board of scientific advisers of the National Cancer Institute and is chairperson of the National Consensus Project for Quality Palliative Care. She has authored nine books, including *Cancer Pain Management* (1995), *Suffering* (1996), *Pain in the Elderly* (1996), and the *Oxford Textbook of Palliative Nursing*, published by Oxford University Press (4th ed., 2015). She is co-author of *The Nature of Suffering and the Goals of Nursing* (Oxford University Press, 2008) and *Making Health Care Whole: Integrating Spirituality into Patient Care* (Templeton Press, 2010).

Foundations in palliative and end-of-life care

This is my 37th year as a nurse. I began my career on inpatient oncology, which at the time was really quite new, the idea of chemotherapy, and the idea of having oncology units. The culture around me was all about treating the tumour. From the first day I walked into the oncology unit, my desire was to care for the seriously ill, advanced disease, and dying patient. I really felt my calling to be symptom management, comfort care, explaining to families what was happening, having difficult conversations, advocating for patients and their goals of care, and getting people out of the hospital where possible. During that time, the introduction of the DRG system (diagnostic related groups) was taking root in the US health care system. This was a significant change in American health care because it incentivized hospitals to discharge people home. Prior to that, if you called from home and you said, 'Oh, my husband is having nausea', or 'I think my mother is getting weaker', they would bring you in. All the incentives were to hospitalize people. It seemed to me that almost overnight, the hospitals were saying, We don't need to admit these people; we have to discharge them home. You barely got them in the bed and they were looking to send them home. That astounded me. I thought these people are barely able to cope here in the hospital, even with our support being immediately available to them. How can they manage all of this at home? So, I had this burning interest to see what was happening in home care. After three years of working on inpatient oncology, I went to work with a home care agency. There were no hospices in my state, but many patients being referred for home care really needed hospice. Over the next three years, I actually helped to start the first hospice programme in the state. This was before there was hospice certification, and hospice was still so new.

At the same time, while I was working in the home care agency, I decided to get a master's degree. I felt at times I was banging my head against a brick wall. Patients and families had needs that were not being addressed and I could not get the system to listen to me. I needed data to support what I was saying but I also needed the knowledge, credentials, and tools to change practice. So I went back to school and got a master's degree.

The further I got into this work, I realized that I needed data to support what I was doing and so needed greater research skills, beyond the practice and quality improvement learning I had gained through my master's degree. So, I went back to school again and got my doctorate.

The focus of my doctoral dissertation was home versus hospital cancer death and bereavement outcomes. My hypothesis was that families reluctantly take their loved one home to die, with little preparation, with just a commitment to do what the patient wants. How do they manage that care? What I did see was that when families were able to take their loved one home and provide good care for them, they felt very good about being able to do that, and so I could then consider how that caring impacted their bereavement.

I think that was really the beginning of my career and 37 years later, here I am.

The compassionate practitioner

Because of my work with the end-of-life nursing education project (ELNEC), I have spent 14 years asking how do we prepare nurses to be both compassionate and competent. It is a complicated question. I was really inspired hearing Dame Cicely Saunders comment that people need our compassion, but they also need our competence. I thought that was so true, because I saw a lot of people who were very kind and compassionate, but still did not know what they were doing. They were out there holding people's hands and saying 'I am so sorry' while the person was in agonizing pain.

Alternatively, people were providing technically excellent care, but without an ounce of compassion. Neither is correct. People need excellence in care, while being cared for by professional people. So what comes to my mind is the notion of empathy, and I do believe empathy is a necessary element of compassion. I think we want people to feel empathy, but we want the expression of that empathy to be this broader thing that we call compassion. Empathy is the entrée to compassion. If I take the example of a young mother who is dying and leaving her children behind, I can feel that suffering, perhaps even understand it, and express to that mother how sorry I am that they are going through this and how incredibly difficult it must be. That is my empathetic entrée.

But compassion is more. I can then sit down next to that mother. I am prepared and committed to be present for that mother and to listen to her story, because she is the one who is living it. Presence is a very big component of compassion. Compassion means that I am willing to sit and listen to her tell me what this is like for her and to stay there with her, listen to her, and then respond to her, in a way that goes beyond empathy in a compassionate way.

I think the Henri Nouwen definition very much captures what I was trying to distinguish between empathy and compassion. To me, the phrase 'going where it hurts' (Nouwen et al. 1982: 4) and the notion of sharing and full immersion is very powerful. In the (ELNEC) project, we use a phrase taken from a passage by Nicholas Wolterstorff, talking about the death of this son: 'Come sit beside me on my mourning bench.' You can be kind and shake his hand and say how sorry you are and keep moving. But to bring compassion to life, I would approach this man on his mourning bench. I would extend my hand. I would look into his eyes. I would be very present in my interaction with him; I would express my shared sorrow and the depth of understanding, to the degree that I can have it:

> I have not lost my son, but I have listened to you. I have watched you. I know you are a loving father, so I do have some insight into your suffering and I am expressing my sorrow in sharing your suffering. Let me abide with you today. You have told me this story 14 times and I am here today to hear it again. Maybe today is so overwhelming to you because it is the anniversary of your son's death. Maybe you do not have the emotional energy to tell me the story again, but I would be glad to sit here again in silence, walk with you to his grave—to not say a word but just be with you.

That is compassion. I can enter his world, but I would never want to imply that my experience becomes his experience or that his experience becomes mine. I am the professional outsider, but I can be present to you and I can go beyond the depths of empathy and move to the place of compassion in which I truly go with you, where it hurts. I share in your suffering and I am willing to let go of my barriers, to the extent that I am here today to fully immerse into your experience.

I have spent a good deal of my life over the last 14 years asking myself if I can teach this to people. What I have come to know is that I can put them in a classroom and, given enough time and a few good resources, I can promise to fill people's brains with knowledge, and do that with such precision now, to be confident that it transcends into practice when they go back to the bedside.

It is a totally different endeavour to try to teach nurses compassion. With symptom management, you are either working with a blank slate, with no prior knowledge, or correcting errors in knowledge to improve practice. With aspects of knowledge, we sometimes have some 'undoing' to do. With compassion, we never start with a blank slate. For any nurse before me, seated in the ELNEC course, I try to help this nurse practise compassion, help this nurse understand what will be necessary for her/him to grow into this. They bring themselves to this learning situation and they bring every relationship, family dynamic, loss, pain, and their personal suffering. I am talking to people who have had this experience of trying to be genuine and open in their professional relationships and they have been hurt in that. Being willing to share comes with a price.

Nurses come to ELNEC, often fairly experienced, and have witnessed many deaths that they bring to the course. When we started the ELNEC paediatric programme, we knew we had to spend time listening to the stories where care was not compassionate. Parents were removed from the bedside of children. Children died in agony. Parents were pushed out the door as quickly as possible. Until nurses can really talk about the suffering they have witnessed, until they can talk about the lack of compassionate care, until they can grieve the chronic losses they have experienced as a nurse, we cannot move them to a new place. At best, I think in our two- or three-day ELNEC course, we give people the opportunity to grieve and to really reflect on the kind of care they have provided, and that has been provided around them, and open a few doors about what compassionate care might look like and what they personally need in their continuing development to get to that place of compassionate care.

We often do a very simple listening exercise where we pair people up and the role of one person is to speak of a loss and the role of the second person is to sit silently and listen to an expression of loss. So many times I have heard nurses say, 'I have been a nurse for 18 years and I have never sat silently for five minutes.' This is the practice of compassion, because we are asking them to go where a person is hurting.

Over 14 years, ELNEC has trained over 17,000 nurses, across 78 countries, now who themselves have gone on to train about 400,000 people. ELNEC creates a space for nurses who experience a level of discomfort with practice and are saying, 'I think there is a better way.' ELNEC offers that space to recognize what is missing, what compassionate care could be, and we send them home with a new network of people and support, in the knowledge that they will grow into the role of the ELNEC-trained nurse—which I think in many ways is the same as saying, a compassionate practitioner.

A case exemplar

The case is one I observed easily 15 years ago now. I was doing a study on pain management at home and working in home care agencies to identify patients who were in home care, with pain problems. Our project was really about helping the nurses do a better job of holistic pain management at home. I had gone to interview a patient with very late stage prostate cancer, with widespread bone metastases. He was an older man, emaciated, bed-bound, totally immobilized by his pathological fractures, and miserable. His wife, who was also elderly, frail, exhausted, and overwhelmed, was caring for him for. I started into my interview but personally, I was just taken by the degree of pain and suffering this man was enduring.

The hospice nurse came into the room. She was a nurse I knew a little, because she had been part of the training in the agency. I told her I could wait and she should take care of him. What I witnessed was profound. In my ignorance, I was thinking, Let's get on with it—fix this, assess the pain, score it, call the doctor, change the drugs. Instead, I stood there and watched this nurse. There was nothing rushed, hurried, or urgent about her behaviour. She moved softly and slowly to the bedside, calm and clear—no flipping through the pocket guide, no grabbing for her phone like I would have been doing. She was so present and focused and she got very close to him and looked directly in his eyes and she laid her hands on him. The very first thing she said was:

'Mr. Smith, your wife tells me you are in terrible pain. I am so sorry. I promise we are going to help you, but before we are going to solve this, I am going to ask you some questions. I am going to need to examine you.'

I would never have done that. I would have just marched over there and started giving orders and poking around—it would have been my agenda. I would have been on a mission about the pain in his belly. This woman was 100 per cent with this man; attentive to him, compassionate, present. She reassured him, she went where he was. The man's pain rating must have been reduced by 50 per cent when she walked in the room. What an incredibly respectful thing that was. She was saying I need your permission and I need you to understand that I do understand you are miserable and suffering, and I am going to do what I have to do, but as quickly as possible, so we can get what you need. He nodded. He understood and trusted her.

She then did an expert physical examination, compassionate and competent, the best physical examination I have seen. It wasn't just about his body. Then she paused, looked at him and said, 'Can you tell me how it feels to you?' This was a wise nurse who knew this pain. We might interpret this pain physically, but he is the man living this. This was profound to the patient—she saw that this pain was not the pain of the ten other people she was seeing that day. The patient said,

It feels as if I have a zipper running down the front of me and it feels as if someone just unzipped me, reached both hands inside of me and grabbed my stomach with both hands and started wringing it dry—that is how it feels.

She replied, 'That sounds horrible, someone reaching inside you, grabbing your stomach and wringing it dry—are you feeling that feeling all the time or does it come and go?' He said, 'I feel the pain all the time, but every time I pee it is a killer.'

This took 30 seconds. In 30 seconds, we knew so much more about this man's experience. It was profound. It was important clinically, because what the nurse figured out was that this man had developed a severe urinary tract infection and was having extreme bladder spasm. She cared enough to go deeply and hear his words and she was so competent in the physical act of her exam, she was getting to the human experience. This is compassion through competence. Through her compassionate questioning, she could obtain insightful, deep understanding.

She could then tell the doctor, 'I am with this man. He is clearly at the end of his life; he is suffering immensely. I believe he is having a severe UTI with extreme bladder spasm and we must respond immediately.' The message she gave was that we are going to deal with this right now, give him the most powerful antibiotic, because he is going to die in the next few days, but not with extreme bladder spasm. We are going to treat that. We are going to add medication to treat the pain. We are going to explain to him and his wife what is happening and we are going to come back later today and tomorrow, until the medicine can begin to work on the bladder spasm. We are going to now do that active palliative care response that really speaks to all that the medical world can offer—that very personal, very attentive response to the real goals of care. It all happened and the man died peacefully a few days later. I have thought about that visit a hundred times or more, and there were so many ways this could have played out, but what that nurse did was no less than a work of art. You could take the 1,200 pages out of my *Oxford Textbook of Palliative Nursing* or you could look at this nurse, because there it was—one nurse practising 'textbook', complete palliative care.

Fostering sustainable compassion

When you ask about compassion today, what you hear is that hospitals are so overburdened, clinics are too crowded, people have only 12 minutes to do a new patient visit, and so on. It is all excuses. I think when people say there is less opportunity for compassion, our care is less compassionate, what they mean is we are busier and have less time. I don't think it is about time. I could share ten stories where I saw compassion in action, and all those interactions took five minutes or less. Of course, it is wonderful when you have the opportunity to sit with someone for 20 minutes, but it is not necessary. Compassion is not about that. Compassion is about who you are, how you approach the patient. People can be compassionate in the midst of total chaos. I have seen some of the best compassion in the poorest, most under-resourced countries. It is almost that when all that you have to offer is yourself, compassion happens. I would disagree with any notion that compassion happens less frequently or is less important today. I would say the total opposite. There has never been a time where our health care system has been more overburdened, frantic, disconnected, and there has never been a time where the people we serve need compassionate care more.

When I was a child we went to our family practice doctor. He did it all. He really did have 30 minutes to talk to you. It was a different time where things moved slower, where there was more time for human interaction. Things have changed. There was a time when people stayed in hospital for ten days, now we see them in the clinic for 20 minutes and send them home. We now have more articulate consumers. We have patients and families who have an expectation that someone needs to tell them what is going on. Professionals have higher skills in communication, empathy, the ability to set goals for care. We manage complex family meetings and care is much less patriarchal than it used to be. So in terms of the future, I am very hopeful, because I think health care will look incredibly different. I think people who are entering health care do so because they are seeking meaningful work. People are becoming clinicians because they personally seek an opportunity for a human connection to release suffering, to be compassionate people. I am very encouraged. I think we have learned some things about how to promote compassionate values. I am very interested in the idea of what you need to be a palliative care provider. We all agree if you are going to do this work, you need to be knowledgeable about pain management and psychological issues. You need to have competent skills in family counselling and communications. I am very intrigued with the whole idea about the spirituality of the provider. The nurse that I described in the case had a very strong Buddhist practice. I think her Buddhist practice was evident in her compassionate approach.

I co-chair the National Clinical Practice Guidelines of Palliative Care, which has eight domains, one of which is spirituality. We talk in the guidelines about the skill required for proficiency. So what does it mean to say you have to be spiritually proficient to work in palliative care? We are not saying that everyone who works in palliative care has to take on a formal religious tradition, but I do think many people would contend it is very hard to be compassionate and empathetic unless you practice self-care and have some insight into yourself as a person. There are many guidelines that say to be a palliative care provider you need to have some spiritual practice of your own. Whether that is taking a walk three times a week in nature because of a connection with the universe and nature, or through meditation, yoga, poetry, or some form of prayer. I do think it is the missing piece. I think you can be with people who are seriously ill and dying and you can have great communication skills, great cultural awareness, and know a lot about empathy, but if you don't have some sense of your own spirituality or spiritual practice, I think it is very difficult to be a compassionate provider. I think in our increasingly diverse society, we care daily for people from diverse faith backgrounds. For me, compassion goes beyond religion, although I do think it is very important to understand the place of compassion across all religious traditions. I have expressed that often and I am always asked if I am saying that an atheist cannot be a hospice nurse. I am quick to say that people without a faith tradition can be superb providers of palliative care, but I do think everyone needs some aspect of spirituality in their lives.

Commentary

Betty Ferrell's explanation of the 'empathic entrée' and her distinction between that and compassion alludes to the fact that, unquestionably, the literature on compassion is controversial. Compassion has been explored from many scientific, sociological, psychological, and anthropological perspectives, particularly with regard to its relationship to similar states, such as pity, sympathy, love, and empathy (Nussbaum 1996; Ekman 2003; Sprecher & Fehr 2005). Goetz et al. (2010) choose to place these states in a familial relationship to compassion but argue that compassion itself is a 'distinct affective experience' (p. 351). The relationship between empathy and compassion is equally complex. Svenaeus (2014) proposes that empathy is central to medicine by virtue of its being the 'feeling component' (p. 247) of *phronesis*—the Aristotelian concept of 'practical wisdom'. Further, empathy presupposes a mutual engagement between the professional and the patient (Halpern 2014). In this way, the suffering of the other (the patient) can be felt by me (the professional) and therefore approached and managed appropriately. Others, such as Cindy Wigglesworth, a US-based corporate leadership consultant, would support Betty Ferrell's assertion that empathy precedes compassion, and offers a framework to explain that (Wigglesworth 2012). In brief, the difference between empathy and compassion is that whereas empathy enables us to feel what the sufferer is feeling in a genuine and caring way, compassion enables us to do the same thing but without becoming overwhelmed by the other's suffering, enabling the practitioner to be fully present and able to act skilfully and meaningfully. For the field of palliative and end-of-life care, the idea of 'exquisite empathy', first studied by Harrison and Westwood (2009) with practitioners working with traumatized clients, has gained increased recognition, notably in relation to physician caregiving at end of life (Kearney et al. 2009). *Exquisite empathy* requires the practitioner to be able to create an intimate and meaningful connection with the patient or client, whilst at the same time being able to maintain professional perspective. This approach offers a practical orientation to the clinician needing to engage at a deeper level and enables the innate human context of compassion to become concrete. Moreover, utilizing an approach such as this can enhance the quality of interaction without the burden of strain and burnout that has become so commonplace in the vernacular of health care today (Renzenbrink 2011). What seems key to this is the place of some inner work or practice, which enables the practitioner to engage the heart and mind in a meaningful and soulful way.

Reflections for practice

+ What strikes you most about the approach of the hospice nurse in the case presented by Betty Ferrell?
+ Which of the traits presented in her practice do you find most challenging?
+ If there are risks to engaging compassionately with patients, such as compassion fatigue and/or burnout, what supportive practices can you create to avoid being overwhelmed?

Further reading

Ekman P (2003) Emotions revealed: recognizing faces and feelings to improve communication and emotional life. New York: Henry Holt.

Ferrell BR, Ferrell William Ed, Ferrell William Ed (1996) Pod-Suffering: Human dimensions Pain/Illness. Burlington, Jones and Bartlett Learning.

Ferrell BR, Ferrell BA (1996) Pain in the elderly: task for on pain in the elderly. Baltimore, IASP Press.

Ferrell BR, Coyne, N (2008) The nature of suffering and the goals of nursing. Oxford, Open University Press.

Goetz JL, Keltner D, Simon-Thomas E (2010) Compassion: an evolutionary analysis and empirical review. Psychological Bulletin, **136**(3), 351–374.

Halpern J (2014) From idealized clinical empathy to empathic communication in medical care. Medicine, Health Care and Philosophy, **17**(2), 301–311.

Harrison R, Westwood M (2009) Preventing vicarious traumatization of mental health therapists: identifying protective practices. Psychotherapy, Theory, Research, Practical Training, **46**(2), 203–219.

Kearney MK, Weininger RB, Vachon MLS, Mount BM, Harrison RL (2009) Self-care of physicians caring for patients at the end of life: 'being connected . . . a key to my survival'. Journal of the American Medical Association, **301**, 1155–1164.

Nussbaum MC (1996) Compassion: the basic social emotion. Social Philosophy and Policy, **13**, 27–58.

Pulchalski C, Ferrell B (2010) Making health care whole: integrating spirituality into patient care. Philadelphia, Templeton Press.

Sprecher S, Fehr B (2005) Compassionate love for close others and humanity. Journal of Social and Personal Relationships, **22**, 629–651.

Svenaeus F (2014) The phenomenology of empathy in medicine: an introduction. Medicine, Health Care and Philosophy, **17**, 245–248.

Wigglesworth C (2012) SQ21: the twenty-one skills of spiritual intelligence. New York, Selectbooks

Wolterstorff N (2002) Lament for a son. The Living Pulpit, October-December, 13.

Chapter 11

Kathy Foley—The Golden Rule

Dr Kathleen M. Foley is an attending neurologist in the Pain and Palliative Care Service at Memorial Sloan Kettering Cancer Center in New York City. She is also professor of neurology, neuroscience, and clinical pharmacology at Weill Medical College of Cornell University, and previous director of the WHO Collaborating Center for Cancer Pain Research and Education at Memorial Sloan Kettering Cancer Center. Her career has focused on the assessment and treatment of patients with cancer pain. With her colleagues, she has developed scientific guidelines for the use of analgesic drug therapy through clinic pharmacologic studies of opioid drugs.

Kathy Foley holds the chair of the Society of Memorial Sloan Kettering Cancer Center in Pain Research. She was elected to the Institute of Medicine of the National Academy of Sciences for her national and international efforts in the treatment of patients with cancer pain. She is past director of the Open Society Foundations Project on Death in America, whose goal was to transform the culture of dying in the United States through initiatives in research, scholarship, and clinical care.

She has received numerous awards, including the Medal of Honor from the American Cancer Society, the David Karnovsky Award from American Society of Clinical Oncology, and the Frank Netter Award from the American Academy of Neurology. She also chaired three expert committees that resulted in the publication of the three seminal WHO monographs on cancer pain and palliative care: *Cancer Pain Relief* (1986), *Cancer Pain Relief and Palliative Care* (1990), and *Cancer Pain and Palliative Care in Children* (1996).

She is currently the medical director of the International Palliative Care Initiative of the Open Society Public Health Program, working to advance palliative care globally.

Foundations in palliative and end-of-life care

I trained as a neurologist and came to Memorial Sloan Kettering Cancer Center (MSKCC) in 1974 to do a special fellowship in neuro-oncology. I became an attending physician in 1975. I came here to develop a clinical research programme in pain in cancer patients. There was a funding source for rehabilitation medicine to develop a clinical pain programme and I came to join a team who had, at that point, a very well-established analgesic study group. My role was to try to understand the nature of pain in patients with cancer, since pain was considered one of the neurological complications of cancer due to its clear manifestation through the nervous system. No one knew anything about pain in patients with cancer. At that time in this institution, pain management was relatively poor, with most patients getting injectable drugs on a p.r.n or 4–6 hourly basis. Yet there was a great deal of expertise here on how to assess new analgesic agents and how to measure pain.

In 1981, we established the first pain clinic in a cancer centre in the US and then, in the mid-80s, we developed the Supportive Care Program, because the word hospice or palliative care was not something easily understood or accepted here by either patients and families or professionals. In the mid-90s, we changed the name of the service to the Pain and Palliative Care Service. I must say that I felt a little bit dragged into palliative care, because my focus was on the care of cancer patients who were receiving active therapy, including the care of patients who were dying. Eighty per cent of our referrals were patients with advanced illness, and 75 per cent of our patients died within three months of consultation. It took time to evolve understanding about the critical importance of pain management in patients with very advanced illness. It became very apparent that we needed to attend to much more than simply their pain because their suffering was profound and related to so many other factors. In the last year, the name of the service has now changed again to the Palliative Care Service.

I think there are different interpretations on how we discuss palliative care from the North American perspective. If you view the North American approach being that of Balfour Mount's Canadian hospital consultancy service, then we adopted that within MSKCC. We developed a WHO collaborating centre in pain research and education, so the language of palliative care was integral to how we thought about the kind of care we needed to deliver to cancer patients and used this to frame the cancer control programme approach.

In 1993 a social worker, Patricia Prem, brought together a group of people to advise her friend the philanthropist George Soros on how we might improve the care of the dying in the US. She had worked with patients with advanced renal disease and was very sensitive to the issues of end-of-life care. After several months of national consultation, a meeting was arranged at George Soros's home with a wide range of different experts from hospice, the law, pain management, palliative care, and cancer. Soros offered $15 million to fund projects to improve the care of the dying. That eventually evolved into The Project on Death in America. We rapidly appointed a board; I became the director of that project. We named it The Project on Death in America because we thought it was important to put the word *death* in the name of the project to try to expand and increase conversations around the topic. Over a nine-year period, we spent $45 million to fund US activities to improve the care of the dying. David Clark (2013) has published a book about it called *Transforming the Culture of Dying: The Work of The Project on Death in America*.

Whenever you begin a project that is so different, you clearly cannot know what the outcomes might be, but the project exceeded much more than we could have ever anticipated. Going into the project, we understood some of the levers of power that needed to change to improve the care of the dying and we focused on those levers. We identified that the way to change medicine was from within. So we needed champions to lead palliative care into its next stage of development. We supported individual champions—doctors, nurses, social workers. It was incredibly good fortune that at the same time we were developing this initiative, the Robert Wood Johnson Foundation was developing their public health programmes and they put another $250 million into the field. We had this wonderful synergy with a very large, powerful health foundation thinking this was an important topic and we, who were more innovative and catalytic, could start projects that they could take to scale.

So in terms of outcomes, palliative medicine became a speciality, the individuals who were part of our faculty scholars and leadership programmes became the leaders in the field, the editors of the journals, the professors of medicine. Today they direct some of the 70 different fellowship programmes that exist in the country. I think we transformed medicine from within with those leaders and we partially influenced public policy, predominantly in the area of cancer. In 2001, I edited a report for the Institute of Medicine called 'Improving Palliative Care for Cancer' which basically said we were not doing much. Today, we have a total transformation—the American Society of Clinical Oncology views palliative care as one of its important and essential roles.

The compassionate practitioner

Compassion means being a good doctor. Nothing more, nothing less. For the most part, I am not sure that doctors want that term applied to them because they want to be seen as competent, and compassion can be the trade-off—well, they are compassionate, but that is not the same as competent. I think there is sometimes a tension that physicians see in using language that is more emotionally than scientifically laden. There is a strong pragmatic element to compassion. You need to answer the patients' phone calls; you need to be able to respond to their questions quickly; you need to facilitate their care; you need to advocate for them. In all of that you have to have the equanimity to know where you are going and that you are going to get them there. It is critically important to acknowledge what you know and don't know and encourage rather than limit consultation. So I think therein lie the issues. There are qualities that need to happen, but at heart, compassion should be the essence of a good doctor.

The Nouwen definition is beautifully phrased but I think it is more about the impact on the clinician than the person. It is a somewhat narcissistic definition of compassion because it focuses on where *we* have to go as opposed to where the patient may be. It seems more inward-looking. The definition is about an understanding of sharing in the brokenness of people that we are ministering to, as well as ourselves. I love the component that it requires 'full immersion in the condition of being human'; one human caring for another human being (Nouwen et al. 1982: 4). This requires us to clearly know the patient as well as we need to know their disease and be detailed and accurate about their disease and how it influences their life. Several years ago, Dr Nathan Cherny, a fellow here, Nessa Coyle, a PhD nurse who directed our supportive care programme, and I put together a paper calling for a taxonomy of suffering on how we approach our patients. We focused on identifying the physical, psychological, social, and existential needs of our patients and their families. This whole concept of treating their suffering was based on our perspective that we were trying to be compassionate and competent physicians. We needed to understand people's fears and anxieties and more globally; we needed to understand their suffering.

I have wrestled with the question of whether faith is important for compassion because I don't know if I have enough insight into myself to be able to answer that. I clearly have a faith. It seems to me that the care of those who suffer is quite universal. This particular definition is not very different to what Eric Cassell says about suffering, or agnostic views of suffering. I edited a book with a psychiatrist colleague who would identify himself as an agnostic, yet this isn't a definition he would find difficult to embrace. I think it is all about humanism here. This seems quite a humanistic definition that would fit with a perspective of social justice. The respect for the condition of being human comes from a human rights perspective—the dignity of the individual.

How I separate my everyday practice from my faith base is always a dilemma for me because I function in such a secular world and I am a little bit protective of that faith component. I respect the moral value and being of the individual but I don't find that particularly religious. It is not that faith may be important. It is just that I have not been able to parse out what it is and is not.

There is always a debate about whether we can teach compassion. We have wonderful discussions about why we can't teach empathy but we can teach empathetic behaviour. I would say we *can* teach compassion; that is, we can teach people what it is; we can name it; we can describe it and we can show practices related to it. As one can do that, it should be amenable to teaching. Probably the most important role we play is to model compassion. There was an interesting series of papers published in the *New York Times* about raising a moral child. They reported on a series of experiments which demonstrated that a compassionate act by a teacher or role model was much more influential than anything they said to a child. So it is the power of modelling behaviour. Medicine is so socialized in the way that we practice, in the kind of professionalism that we engage in, the sort of rules that we accept. Since so much of medicine is based on mentorship and on role model behaviour, one would think you could role model compassionate behaviours so it becomes the norm. Less than the norm then becomes unacceptable as part of the culture.

A case exemplar

I cared for a young man who was a third-year resident physician in another institution. Peter was diagnosed with an advanced osteosarcoma. He came back to where his family lived. Unfortunately, widely metastatic disease was confirmed, and his tumour had spread to his lungs and other lymph nodes throughout his body. He was reeling from being both a doctor and a patient with this diagnosis. As soon as he would finish his bout of chemotherapy, he would drag himself from his bed and go back to work in a student health clinic at one of our local universities, teaching medical students who rotated through the clinic with him. To my mind, you witness the most extraordinary degree of compassion from this college who supported him to continue seeing these college students on a regular basis. He had no hair and looked sick and could hardly walk about in the clinic. He modelled this extraordinary level of care to these college students but also to the medical students about how to assess their fellow students and how to talk to them about their lives and how to understand their current medical illnesses.

When Peter subsequently died, it was discovered that he had left a reflective diary on his entire illness. We did not know he was keeping this diary. It took me back a bit. It was the immense realization that you don't know who your patients are; you don't know what they are thinking or why they act as they do. It was extraordinarily humbling.

During the time he was under our care he had also agreed to participate in a film called *Doctors with Cancer*. We had this extraordinary diary information and all the outtakes for the film we had made with him. A wonderfully creative producer friend of mine decided to put them together as a video where you see how the director of the clinic let this young man be a functioning doctor within that clinic, let him live his life as fully as possible. The compassion that this individual showed to enable that, not to mention the courage of that system which allowed him to be there when he was so fragile and sick, honouring who he was, and not what he was at that moment. You can only imagine the paperwork that came with that. When Peter was alive, the medical students were interviewed and asked what they thought about him and each one spoke about both his compassion and competence and what they learnt from him. It created an environment which enabled this incredibly vulnerable individual to give back to the profession that we all have such respect for.

Fostering sustainable compassion

I think systems can create an environment for compassionate care but I don't think we can really have compassionate care unless each person accepts their individual responsibility in that. The ethos of the institution must acknowledge that we provide humane compassionate care. You need a welcoming environment and you need someone who is willing to provide that care. I have no reason to think those who enter the field of medicine don't have a degree of compassion or see their role is to treat suffering. First, you need to find the environment that allows you to express that and to stay away from environments that do not appreciate it, or, alternatively, try to change them. You need to select out the environments that match your personality as well as your personal and professional goals.

The second thing is that medicine is a science so that you have to be really good at what you do from a scientific perspective. You cannot be compassionate and *sort of* a good doctor; you have to be a *great* doctor who is also compassionate. Then those systems need to be in place: systems that honour and respect the individual, are flexible in design, and have adopted the hotel industry perspective in terms of welcome and service. We need protocols so that if the right level of compassionate care is not delivered, we have a way to challenge that, but more importantly, to improve it. We need to start this with very simple principles such as making pain a fifth vital sign as we have done throughout the US. If we don't measure and document it, we won't talk about it. In the same way, measuring and reporting distress leads to a protocol for assessing distress which can be shared with other members of the team. We need the full range of services for it to be a real palliative care service and I would particularly note social worker and chaplaincy services here. The reason I identity those in particular is because of the breadth of physical, social, and existential dimensions which need to be attended to.

This is a tall order in settings that are already anxiety-laden and have to manage an extraordinary amount of fear and concern on the part of patients and families who can easily act out and attack anyone who stands in their way. In a demanding and complex system, the level of tone set is all-important; not just the doctor or nurse but from the very first person they meet at the front desk. It is at every stage.

I remember a study undertaken here by Dr Nathan Cherny, where it was basically suggested that physicians were neither compassionate nor competent in how they delivered pain management to patients. The head of the surgical department said, 'Well, the fish rots from the top', so we have to start there and you need leadership that is open to this.

Translating a message of palliative care as social justice for the future really depends on where the next generation of practitioners will live. In highly developed countries, we have had such advances in protecting the rights of individuals that we don't see human rights in the same framework that we might see in a less developed country. For example, in the US we have a patients' bill of rights. Patients have the right to receive information, to refuse treatment, the right to question their doctor, and they have the right to pain treatment. It has become such a part of the fabric of our system that it is a given. However, we still see the need for attention to justice in the inequalities and disparities in care that is delivered. In the US, patients who are Hispanic or African American are consistently under-medicated for their pain because of their ethnicity. Patients who are financed through our Medicaid health system do not necessarily receive medical care in a timely fashion or in a fashion that provides them with continuity of care and attention to assist the full spectrum of their needs. There are clearly gaps to be addressed.

If you look at this from the perspective of a low-resource country, the human rights piece is critically important. What they need to demand is that their government respect the WHO mandate that essential medicines should be a part of the right to health care. The social justice argument is framed by respect for the dignity of the individual and understanding how we apply human rights within a bioethics framework to the care that we deliver to them. However, decision-makers won't hear this argument if civil society does not ask for it and if civil society does not know that they have a right to this, how could they begin to demand it? The patients and families that we care for are so consumed with trying to get the care they need, they can't begin to advocate for something beyond that, and they don't know there is something better. They don't know that their pain could be treated. They don't know that their distress can be managed. They don't know that there are social supports that might make a difference. They have never died so how can they know what is it like to die? They don't know that needless suffering could be ameliorated. This is all in the framework of their not wanting to talk about this part of their life. That is why it is so important for the palliative care profession to lead civil society to find their voice and begin to say, 'I have the right to this.'

I think there has been a sea change of activities over the last 25 years, partially driven by the concept of professionalism. When our health care industry, specifically the physicians, are accused of being part of the marketplace economy, the reaction to that has been that we need to reclaim our professionalism. Learning around professionalism is now mandated within US medical residency training, including the number of hours to be spent on it and greater focus on how to use and engage the humanities. I would say with the rise of bioethics in this country, there has been a great deal more attention to what defines and describes those professional activities. With the focus on caring for the dying, increasing attention is placed on how important it is for physicians to address the whole-person suffering of their patients, not just their physical distress but their psychosocial and existential distress as well. With the expansion of the field of palliative care, there is so much more attention needed on how to communicate what this care can mean to the whole person and their family. In no way do I think that palliative medicine is going to save the rest of medicine, but I do think it is going to model the care, for those in a way are the most vulnerable in the system because of their advanced illness.

Commentary

In the case for the Charter for Compassion (http://www.charterforcompassion. org), the author and theologian Karen Armstrong takes as her starting point the need for us to reclaim the Golden Rule. First cited by Kongfuxi (Confucius) five centuries before Christ, his adage 'Do not impose on others what you do not wish for yourself' (Freedman 2002) resonates with the spirit of compassion and reflects the core philosophy of all the major religions of the world. Put another way, Confucius argued that to live the Golden Rule meant that 'you leave yourself behind, you dethrone yourself from your world and put another there, you achieve transcendence from selfishness, and that is what God is' (Freedman 2002). Karen Armstrong's more contemporary reflection suggests that the Golden Rule begins with a deep reflection of ourselves before we can really seek to reach out to help others: 'Look into your own heart, discover what it is that gives you pain, and then refuse, under any circumstance whatsoever, to inflict that pain on anybody else' (Armstrong 2009).

We may consider the heart as the seat of compassion. Christina Feldman (2005) suggests that looking into your heart is about commitment and contribution—commitment to end sorrow and willingness to contribute to ease suffering for all beings. Therefore, compassion is not just what we feel, but how we understand, what that feeling means for us, and why it is important that we take action so that others do not suffer in the same way.

We see two constituent elements of compassion demonstrated in this chapter by Kathy Foley which exemplify the notion that compassion is about transforming the world as much as ourselves. Taking the powerful case presented here as an example, the first element respects the individual in their compassionate response to the suffering other; the clinic director towards Peter enabling him to gain enrichment from his professional life to its fullest despite all the challenges that this may pose to him as an administrator. In *The Interior Castle*, the Christian mystic Teresa of Avila proposes that our every action brings the compassion of Christ towards the world, often expressed in the quotation below. This resonates with Peter's own compassionate spirit towards the medical students and university students he cared for in providing a physical witness to compassionate caregiving and the messages he left both them and his professional caregivers by his courage and tenacity: 'Christ has no body now on earth but yours, no hands but yours, no feet but yours. Yours are the eyes through which to look out Christ's compassion to the world' (see Howell 2009).

The second element of compassion reflects how society can nurture or indeed negate the place of compassion. In this chapter, a university takes the courageous step to support Peter to be the person he needed to be at the time when he needed compassion most. As David Clark (2013) asserts in his critical review of The Project on Death in America, compassion is also about responding to a challenge and for those who responded to that challenge, such as Kathy Foley, the impact was immutable. Across communities in America, there are still challenges to the way in which palliative care is delivered (Morrison 2013), but the story which unfolds in this book is one of vision, energy, and, ultimately, compassion. The same can be said of Peter in his story (Chabner 1997).

The first-century Buddhist text *Lotus Sutra* has the power of boundless compassion as its central theme. Feldman (2005) describes this as 'the expression of a liberated heart' (p. 7). This is reflective of the spirit of true generosity which is an essential component of the cultivation of compassion (Karzan 2013). Compassion is expansive and through its practice we extend compassion to all sentient beings. The message of palliative care as social justice is one of the most visible expressions of universal compassion. The translation of the *Lotus Sutra* into Chinese brought the name *Kuan Yin*—sometimes called the goddess of mercy and compassion—to the fore. The literal translation is 'one who hears the cries of the world' (Feldman 2005). A social justice perspective on palliative care is just that. Reaching out to the world means understanding that compassion is not about power and hierarchy; but sadly, it needs to be envisioned in a world where such things hold importance for the way society is structured. Perhaps if we can re-embrace the Golden Rule as Karen Armstrong hopes we will, then transforming the world to a place of compassion is not beyond the realm of possibility.

Reflections for practice

- To what extent have you seen the principles of the Golden Rule applied to palliative and end-of-life care practice?
- How does the Golden Rule speak to your professional role and discipline practice?
- What messages does Peter's case convey for you in terms of how compassionately we see people living with advanced illness?
- What does it take to transform your world to embrace palliative and end-of-life care more fully?

Further reading

Armstrong K (2009) Let's revive the Golden Rule. TED Global, July. http://www.ted.com/talks/karen_armstrong_let_s_revive_the_golden_rule

Cancer Pain Relief (1986) Geneva WHO Press

Cancer pain relief and palliative care (1990) Geneva, WHO Press.

Cancer pain and palliative care in children (1996) Geneva, WHO Press

Clark D (2013) Transforming the culture of dying: the work of the Project on Death in America. Oxford: Oxford University Press.

Chabner BA (1997) Cancer: a personal journey. Notes from the edge . . . The diary of Peter J. Morgan, MD. Oncologist, 2(4), 206–207.

Cherny N, Coyle N, Foley KM (1994) Suffering in the advanced cancer patient: a definition and taxonomy. Journal of Palliative Care, 10(2), 57–70.

Feldman C (2005) Compassion: listening to the cries of the world. Berkeley, CA: Rodmell.

Freedman R (2002) Confucius: The Golden Rule. Singapore: Scholastic Press.

Howell JC (2009) Introducing Christianity: exploring the Bible, faith and life (1st ed.) Louisville, KY: Westminster John Knox Press.

Karzan B (2013) Cultivating alternative paths to compassion: generosity, forgiveness and patience. In T Singer, M Bolz (eds) Compassion: bridging practice and science. Munich: Max Planck Society.137–157.

Morrison RS (2013) Models of palliative care delivery in the United States. Current Opinion in Supportive and Palliative Care, 7(2), 201–206.

St Teresa of Avila (2010) The interior castle (study ed.; transl. K Kavanaugh, O Rodriguez). Washington: ICS.

Chapter 12

Charles von Gunten—
The truth of time

Dr Charles F. von Gunten received a BA with honours from Brown University in Providence, Rhode Island, in 1978. He then earned a PhD in biochemistry and an MD degree with honours from the University of Colorado Health Sciences Center in Denver, Colorado, in 1988. He subsequently pursued residency training in internal medicine, followed by sub-specialty training in haematology/oncology at the McGaw Medical Center of Northwestern University in Chicago. As assistant professor of medicine at Northwestern University Medical School until 1999, he directed programmes in hospice and palliative care, education, and research. Until recently, he was clinical professor of medicine at University of California, San Diego, where he was a member of the NIH-designated Moores Comprehensive Cancer Center. In addition he was the provost, Institute for Palliative Medicine at San Diego Hospice, a teaching and research affiliate of the University of California, San Diego, and San Diego State University.

In 2012, he moved to Columbus, Ohio, to become Vice President, Medical Affairs, Hospice and Palliative Medicine for the Ohio health system. He has held an established investigator award from the National Cancer Institute and is the editor-in-chief of the *Journal of Palliative Medicine*. In 2013, the American Academy of Hospice and Palliative Medicine voted him amongst the ten top 'visionaries' in palliative medicine today.

He has a particular interest in the integration of hospice and palliative care into academic medicine and has published and spoken widely on the subjects of hospice, palliative medicine, and pain and symptom control.

Foundations in palliative and end-of-life care

My first step was when I was in medical school and a friend of mine was a volunteer chaplain in a local hospice. He told me about an elderly woman who was convinced she was deposed royalty from Europe. She was being 'held' in this nursing home, made to wear these dreadful gowns that did not befit a person of her rank, and was not treated with the respect due to someone of noble breeding. Staff saw her as a problem. She was disruptive; she threw food and they wanted her medicated. My friend said he went to the local thrift store and bought some lovely peignoirs lined with caribou fur and some lace for a few dollars and gave them to her. Her behaviour changed because she felt recognized, and she had a happy course thereafter. That was intriguing to me because that was not what I was learning in medical school. We had no hospice rotation and so I did two weeks with that particular hospice. When I was in residency training, there was a hospice unit in the hospital and I was asked to provide coverage as part of being an intern. I noticed the care there was different for the same type of patients as I was admitting elsewhere in the hospital. That is what drew me in. It was the quality of the care and approaching people in a different way than I had been taught.

I think in terms of palliative care career opportunity, the US is about 20 years behind the British Isles and Ireland. When I started training, there was no career path in this field. It was never held up as a career for doctors, so I went into oncology. I chose oncology because of the intensity of the relationships with patients and family. When someone has cancer there is no small talk. When the doctor walks in the room, the only barrier to talking about the most profound parts of human existence is the willingness of the doctor, the courage of the doctor to be able to talk about it. Patients and their families are right there with you and I like that. So oncology was a good place for me. As my training in oncology came to an end, I had the opportunity to become a hospice medical director. We were just hearing about palliative care services and I had the ability to do that in my hospital and it took off from there.

I am now 25 years in palliative medicine, most notably in San Diego. I was recruited there from an academic medical centre to help them build their education and research programmes. It was a free-standing hospice supported by the community. Over 13 years, I had a wonderful time building education programmes for medical students, residents, fellows, community physicians, and nurses. By the time I left, we had 4,000 learners coming to us every year. Our research programme was federally funded, and with a large training programme for specialist physicians, the hospice grew fivefold during that time in terms of the number of people that it was able to serve. I think it is fair to say that we became the most influential hospice in the country over that 13-year period because when you are doing education, research, and outreach, that is really how you bring new ideas. You get everyone galvanized to not just do what they do every day but strive to be the best. I feel firmly that when people, irrespective of discipline, are engaged in teaching and research every day, you are challenged to think, Why am I doing it this way? Is there a better way to be doing it? That is the engine for excellence.

The compassionate practitioner

I think of compassion as my being able to be completely in the present moment with a patient or family member. I try to look through their eyes, with their set of feelings about the current circumstances. What I need to do as a clinician is to silence what is going on in my head; to stop feeling time-pressured, to be fully present with whatever the emotions and feelings are of the patient and family. When those are unhappy, angry feelings, or difficult circumstances that I could never have imagined myself coping with, I need to suspend any kind of analysis in my head, just to be completely present—that to me is being compassionate; to feel with whatever is going on.

I think that the Nouwen definition is accurate—'being with someone when it hurts' (Nouwen et al. 1982: 4)—but I would also say that it is not just those negative perceptions. One of the great pleasures of being in this field is that you are exposed directly to some of the best features of human nature, like love, bravery, courage—you see that routinely every day in people you could never imagine could see it. You can read about these things in books and novels and yet, particularly in advanced disease, it is right there in front of you. I wonder about the idea of 'full immersion'. I would say immersion is more like empathy and compassion is different. Immersion means you lose the position of being able to be therapeutic or helpful because you become one with the person. You lose yourself in their experiences and then you stop being a separate individual. That is where therapeutic misadventures happen—where you agree things are so helpless and hopeless that euthanasia makes sense, or you are so carried away by all the happy thoughts that you really aren't looking ahead and saying, ('Wait a minute, we are heading towards a cliff here.'). To me the compassionate clinician is able to engage with that but without becoming immersed, without becoming lost in the feelings. The privilege of being the clinician is that you are given access to all this but the responsibility is to not lose yourself in it and still be therapeutic. It takes enormous skill and humility to know what is helpful and what is not.

Teaching, at least in health care professions, is less about reading than about experiencing. I firmly believe that all the health professions continue to learn through apprenticeship. The only way anyone learns to be at all helpful is by doing, and you begin at the bottom of that apprenticeship ladder. You just show up and watch and then little by little you are influenced by whom and what you see and you get asked to do. I would say the first step is that the person who wants to learn compassion needs to work with someone who is compassionate. You participate in it, then over time you get to play the role of the compassionate practitioner, but there is somebody else alongside who prevents you from getting lost or immersed, who helps you learn that balance and the exquisite pleasure of being invited into that intimate space of a compassionate relationship. I think there are enormous challenges coming into palliative care. They may think they have the capacity for compassion because of one case or because of a family experience. To be fully present to one tragedy after another takes an emotional hardiness that only comes from experience and enormous support. I can say that people have learnt how to be a compassionate clinician from me. No one ever comes as a blank slate. They are already adults, so who they are is already well established. Shaping, moulding, bringing out characteristics is all part of the teaching environment, but you need a nugget and I think the nugget is just being human. I think human beings are inherently, innately compassionate: you watch it in the nursery; you watch it in the playground. People have enormous innate capacity for compassion.

What separates the teacher from the clinical expert is that you can unpack the experience, pull it apart into its component parts, and be able to make the steps clear to the novice. For example, someone may shadow me at a complex clinical interview and after an hour everybody hugs and has tears and it all seems well done. The trainee says, 'That was wonderful; how did you do that?' As a teacher, I have to pull it apart. How did I walk in? What words did I use? What did you notice when I said this . . . when they said that? A particular facial feature—how I read that. A novice, by definition, can't pull it apart and just do it. Here, you need more than the apprenticeship model can offer, and certainly in medicine and nursing in America, it is not apprenticeship, it is survival. You would wonder if it is truly possible to be compassionate with patients and families and not compassionate with the people you work with. I think this is incredibly important.

A case exemplar

I get asked to see difficult cases, and I was called to see a man from a very prominent family. He was in his middle-80s, living at home with advanced heart failure, advanced emphysema and renal failure which required dialysis. He was rather a cross, grumpy man and although his family were eager for help, his wife was so anxious for me both to understand her fears and where his illness seemed to be taking him, she interviewed me several times to have me understand her husband better. He was basically a scary person! She was anxious that calling me in might have made it all worse. So we had to figure out how she was going to explain to him why I was coming without making him more irritable. We said that there was this new doctor in town who was a very important corporate vice president working to develop programmes for people like her husband and I had heard of him and would be interested to come and see him so I could learn something about his illness and I might be able to offer something. That was all very carefully rehearsed.

It is fairly classic for a patient to react poorly to an interaction with a new physician. I met them both at their home, sitting quietly and trying to see the current situation through his eyes without being affected by his demeanour. Behind the grumpiness and the yelling, I could see an incredibly smart man who was irritated by people not believing him or discounting him because he looked like a wizened caricature of who he used to be. He had trouble getting from bed to chair, but he wanted his dignity, he wanted his sense of control. He knew he was losing that and he was frightened. His wife loved him and wanted to protect him. They had such classic coping strategies. She liked to talk whereas he felt talking made it worse. It was no wonder they felt such distress.

He gradually showed me some of his sense of humour. He knew he was grumpy and pushing people away. He did not like it because he wanted a sense of companionship but did not seem able to help it. He did not want to talk but liked having his wife around. It turned out just facilitating that conversation, in being able to be truly just present, he relaxed, his wife relaxed. There is a sense of timelessness when it happens. I felt so privileged to be pulled into this intimacy. The subsequent meeting was even warmer and we agreed that we would get a physical therapist out to work on his exercise tolerance and that it would be someone that I would hand-pick who would have the ability to work with him. I needed to make sure that the therapist knew that, in this case, this is not the standard come-in-for-your- five-treatments-and-leave. We needed to build this relationship over months, and he needed the companionship. Although he was eligible for hospice care he could not even tolerate talking about that.

I think the key here was to try to not be too controlling. I knew what I wanted him to do but he may not have been willing to do it. I had a strong sense that I was there in large part for the wife, even though he was the one that was sick. The thing that struck me most was their isolation. They were a wealthy family living in a large home in the middle of a forest which just exemplified the isolation. For him, his wife was everything he needed. She needed people and outside contact. In her helplessness, my just showing up was enormous to her and it turned out for him that he was surprised just how much he liked it.

I do think being a man and a doctor shapes the way people treat me. There is no question that it is an advantage. I have frequently been asked to get involved with a patient exhibiting angry or abusive behaviour. I learnt a long time ago it is important to look like a doctor. It is important that I wear a coat and tie. It is important that I carry a little black bag and when I walk in even the most disagreeable person knows what the appropriate behaviour is around a doctor. There clearly is an advantage. It is important that the professional who was experiencing the difficulty is present and we debrief afterwards because it affords an opportunity to provide teaching and guidance around inappropriate professional behaviours or responses that may have led to the anger or abuse. Perhaps if they try some of the things that I say or do it turns out the outcomes are different. It helps manage a situation which may be otherwise just overwhelming and lead to everything that is the exact opposite of compassion.

Fostering sustainable compassion

As an American looking through the lens of American medicine, we have an extraordinary consumerist, business-oriented approach to health care. As in all business, you need to count your outputs and try to maximize productivity per unit cost so outputs are increased. So, you count. You count the procedures, you count the pillows, you count the number of tests, you count how many body systems you have assessed, you count whether various tools have been applied. However, we don't have a way to count compassion, and the conclusion is that quality of compassion and all that goes into it must not be valued. I think it is very important to notice that this conclusion is nobody's real intent. It is an artefact of the focus on counting.

In terms of whether we have lost compassion, I do notice that palliative care clinicians tend to undervalue what they do. They take on the same attitude that the only thing that matters is what you can count and therefore the time I spend is undervalued. By and large, compassion is measured in time given. There is a sort of victim-like quality in terms of 'Oh, they won't give me time.' It comes from a sense that compassion is not valued. What we should be saying is 'This is what I am really good at. I am going to code and bill for all the time I take.'

When I write my documentation I don't only document about the blood pressure I took or the changes in the pain medicine. In the medical record, I clearly, succinctly, and vividly portray the clinical situation with all of its complexities, what we are doing about it, and what the outcome was after the time spent together. There is no rule that nurses, social workers, and chaplains can't write like this. They have just absorbed this from somewhere else, when in fact it is really useful to someone else to say, 'I can't believe that you were in that situation, of course that was a worthwhile amount of time that you spent doing that.'

When I first got into this field I observed the culture of the physicians who wrote in the medical records with a real ink pen, not ballpoint, either a Mont Blanc or Waterman. They always wrote in black ink and about three or four inches in the chart only. Everyone poured over every word afterwards like an orthodox rabbi over the Talmud. I observed that what was different in my notation is that I would use emotional words—'this tragic patient' or 'this inconceivably awful situation'—and then I would write, 'Never before in my career have I ever seen something this difficult.' Nobody ever counts how many times I have written that in the chart. The things we talk about at the nurses' station or in the coffee room between home visits belongs in the medical records where it becomes vivid and observable to everyone else and it also makes it countable. Our mothers told us: 'If you can't say something nice, don't say anything at all.' Documentation reflects that everywhere. People wonder why nobody realizes the difficult things we encounter. You did not speak about it; you did not write about it; you did not make it real. That is what is taking up everybody's time. The patterns in the uniqueness of suffering that you encounter in palliative care are really remarkable.

So compassion is essentially about time. Time is our tests and operations. Time is the thing the rest of the health care systems look for us to do because they don't know how to do it. I can have a compassionate difficult conversation for an hour which makes me no more or less valuable than a surgeon who can spend an hour doing some operation that they know how to do. They are both valuable. Over 25 years, that attitude is what has helped me build the programmes I have and I can point to the clinicians I have trained who similarly do this. We need to value ourselves first.

So for me, compassion is alive and real and is as important now as it ever was in health care. It is deeply valued by patients and families and by our colleagues who ask us to see their patients. Our ability to be compassionate and to be reproducible and reliable in the face of overwhelming tragedy is what distinguishes us as a speciality. Never doubt for a minute that this is what people are asking us for when they ask us to see the person who has pain, or who has a difficult daughter, or who has a sad prognosis. That is what they are asking us for.

Commentary

In this chapter by Charles von Gunten, two critical issues are raised which all palliative care practitioners face in their practice: the expectation and consequences of truth and the meaning and value placed on time.

In *Compassion in Action: Setting Out on a Path of Service*, Ram Dass and Mirabai Bush (1992) contend that

> Compassion is the basis of all truthful relationship: it means being present with love, for ourselves and for all life. . . . Compassion is bringing our deepest truths into our actions, no matter how much the world seems to resist because that is ultimately what we have to give to this world and one another. (p. 5)

At times it can be hard for the patient and family to hear the truth and, as in the case cited here, the reaction can be challenging. The palliative care practitioner may be the visual representation of the truth of what is happening and too painful to accept. The consequences may be withdrawal, rejection, or anger. At the receiving end of that, the practitioner needs some level of self-protection so as not to be overwhelmed by another's suffering. Simple wisdom offered by Charles von Gunten in this chapter such as sitting and listening to the story unfolding and 'trying to look through their eyes' positions us more favourably to be able to extend a compassionate response whatever the circumstance. Further, as demonstrated here, we need to appreciate that an individual's truth may be very different from ours, and somehow we need to accommodate that. There is a significant body of literature on the issue of truth telling which indicates this still remains a crux of debate within health care and, by and large, health care practitioners remain ill-equipped. Rich (2014) argues that 'candid but compassionate communication between physicians and patients about prognosis is essential to informed decisions about both disease-directed (curative) and palliative therapies' (p. 209).

However, he also questions whether the idea of 'terminal' is useful in any discussion that focuses on living well until death, rather than simply 'the dying'. Perget and Lûtzén (2012) conclude that relationship is key to the discourse between patient and clinician, and that even in the most complex circumstance, 'hope must always be inspired' (p. 26). Others, such as de Pentheny O'Kelly et al. (2011), remind us that truth telling is not a 'globally shared moral stance' (p. 3838) but is mediated by both culture and religion. Given this complexity, it would seem important to consider how we prepare ourselves for that engagement in truth. If we move from case to case without any sense of self-reflection on the impact of what has been witnessed in a clinical setting, then we risk losing the professional fulfilment that offering compassionate presence can bring. Consider the way that the discussion regarding documentation about the patient case speaks to the holistic, family-orientated, and person-centred principles that frame the practice of palliative and end-of-life care, and offer a real sense of the living person, rather than the dying patient.

Taking all of these perspectives into consideration, it is evident how the comportment of the physician and the gentle and respectful approach which gives time for adjustment and reconciliation is essential to develop trust, so that when the truth becomes inevitable, the response is always and only compassionate.

In the song 'Only Time', the Irish artist Enya reminds us of a core Buddhist principle—living in the present moment really is the only tangible thing. Beyond that, only time knows. Time is a recurrent theme in this chapter. One of the core skills of the palliative care practitioner is their ability to use time wisely in the pursuit of care, and the ability to offer time is a key indicator for referral from other services. To be able to offer someone who is suffering the sense that your intervention is 'time-less'—not hurried, but fully present to the moment—is expertise that can be nurtured and developed through the apprenticeship approach that is advocated here. One of the earliest experiences for clinicians in understanding the importance of time for patients with advanced disease is the question 'how long have I got?' The nuance of asking this may differ, but it will form a thread of meaning for a patient in their subsequent clinical encounter regarding treatment choices and goals of care. The thoughtful reply to that question affords the clinician an opportunity to explore and express a compassionate response, and in palliative and end-of-life care, practitioners become adept at managing that response in a cogent and supportive way. Learning to be a compassionate practitioner is also something that takes time and speaks to our values and beliefs about the added value of palliative care to the health care experience of the patient and family. A starting point is to stop to consider the phrase 'I wonder . . .' about a situation, a response, or an intervention. Just stopping brings the practitioner back to the present moment so that decisions are always considered and reflective of the situation presented to them. It works.

We cannot change the inevitability of time. His Holiness the Dalai Lama (2011) reminds us that death is inevitable and life cannot be extended beyond its natural course. When death will occur is unknown, but the human lifespan is variable and the body is fragile, so the causes of death are many. Nothing is constant and we all, as human beings, share this one experience. Accepting the impermanence of life does not mean that life is not to be lived. Rather, in the time we have left, there is an onus on those who provide care to ensure that the life of others is lived well and as fully as possible. That is about our compassionate response to both truth and time.

Reflections for practice

- ◆ How do you prepare for encounters where issues of truth are to be discussed?
- ◆ Has there been a time in your practice when stopping for a moment to consider the phrase 'I wonder . . .' would have changed a clinical decision or outcome?
- ◆ Have you considered what the impermanence or inevitability of death means to you? Do you think that is important to explore that idea if you choose to work in a field of practice which involves death and dying?

Further reading

Dass R, Bush M (1992) Compassion in action: setting out on the path of service. New York: Bell Tower.

de Pentheny O'Kelly C, Urch C, Brown EA (2011) The impact of culture and religion on truth telling at end of life. Nephrology Dialysis Transplantation, **26**, 3838–3842.

Dalai Lama (2011) How to be compassionate: a handbook for creating inner peace and a happier world. New York. Atria.

Nouwen HJM, McNeill DP, Morrison DA (1982) Compassion: a reflection on the Christian life. New York: Doubleday.

Perget P, Lűtzén K (2012) Balancing truth-telling in the preservation of hope: a relational ethics approach. Nursing Ethics, **19**(1), 21–29.

Rich BA (2014) Prognosis terminal: truth-telling in the context of end-of-life care. Cambridge Quarterly of Healthcare Ethics, **23**, 209–219.

Chapter 13

Liz Gwyther—Enlightened resolve

Dr Liz Gwyther was born in Zimbabwe and studied medicine at the University of Cape Town, graduating in 1979 with MB ChB. She worked as a GP in Zimbabwe and South Africa and qualified as family physician (FCFP) in 1993. She started in hospice care on a voluntary basis in 1993 and obtained an MSc in palliative medicine from the University of Wales, College of Medicine, in 2003. She is CEO of Hospice Palliative Care Association of South Africa (HPCA) and a director of the following organizations: Networking AIDS Community of South Africa, the African Palliative Care Association, e-hospice, and the Pain Society of South Africa. She is a trustee of the Worldwide Hospice and Palliative Care Alliance (WHPCA).

She is a senior lecturer at the University of Cape Town where she heads the palliative care team within the School of Public Health and Family Medicine. She is the convener for the postgraduate programmes in palliative medicine and is responsible for research supervision and support for publications of the postgraduate students. Her special interests are women's health, palliative care (in particular, palliative care in HIV/AIDS), and human rights in health care. In 2007, she was awarded the SA Medical Association's Gender Award for Human Rights in Health and the SA Institute of Health Managers Leadership in Health Systems award. She is a member of the editorial board of the *Journal of Pain and Symptom Management*.

Foundations in palliative and end-of-life care

My training is as a general practitioner in family practice. One of my classmates at medical school was a mature student called Christine Dare who qualified as a physiotherapist and had worked at St Christopher's Hospice in London. She had spoken to Cicely Saunders about her passion to start a hospice in South Africa. Cicely told her, 'If you want to start a hospice and you want to have people listen to you, you need to qualify as a doctor.' So she started her training the same year that I did and invited Cicely Saunders to a public meeting in our final year at university. So I was sensitized to palliative care and Christine started St Luke's Hospice in Cape Town in 1980.

I worked in quite a rural area about a 90-minute drive out of Cape Town. As a general practitioner, I saw cancer patients whom I referred through to St

Luke's and on one occasion I accompanied one of my patients to St Luke's because Christine was going to initiate her palliative care management, but I was going to continue that management at home as her general practitioner. That was my first step. I then moved into a town practice and when they opened a hospice in Somerset West, which is the eastern suburb of Cape Town, they asked interested general practitioners to do the voluntary back-up for the patients' medical care. Through that role, I attended my first international conference: the Asia Pacific Cancer Conference held in Penang, Malaysia, where Illora Finley was the keynote speaker, and I learnt about the distance learning programme in palliative medicine at Cardiff University.

I qualified with a diploma in palliative medicine and, having promised my family that was the last studying that I was going to do, I received notice that they were starting a master's programme. I enrolled in the master's programme, looking at the need for palliative medicine education in South Africa. Concurrently with my studies, I started the programme at the University of Cape Town which is still the only master's programme in palliative medicine in the continent of Africa. We also have a postgraduate diploma for qualified health care professionals and both programmes are interdisciplinary. We plan to have a throughput of ten students on the master's course and we could enrol more. We had 25 PGD applicants in 2014 and we accepted 23 of them but only 11 enrolled because they could not afford the fees. We had about 19 students on the two-year master's programme.. I am currently doing my PhD which is looking at the South African evidence for palliative care as a human right. Along the way I was employed by the Hospice Palliative Care Association of South Africa in the Education and Training Department and then became the CEO. I have become trustee of the Worldwide Palliative Care Alliance and I manage the Newslink e-hospice South African edition for International News and Views in Palliative Care. Today, I spend 50 per cent of my time with HPCA and 50 per cent of my time is teaching at the University of Cape Town.

The compassionate practitioner

For me, hospice and palliative care means trying to understand and be fully empathetic with the patient and the family member you are looking after. It is truly trying to be patient and family-centred in our care. Trying to understand that empathy is more of an accompaniment of the person, understanding the suffering, without feeling the suffering. The key thing that I try to help our students understand is that if we become overwhelmed by our patients' suffering we can't help them as much as we should. The old teaching of having a professional distance simply does not apply. I think professional distancing gets in the way of compassion. There are strong links here between compassion and palliative care as a human right. I recently presented to our School of Public Health and Family Medicine on dignity as the common foundation of human rights and palliative care, based on Harvey Chochinov's work around the essence of medicine as attitude, behaviour, compassion, and dialogue. Illness can disrupt a person's sense of dignity and compassion is absolutely essential to the professional and empathetic manner which is needed to enhance that dignity. If you read the Universal Declaration of Human Rights (http://www.un.org/en/documents/udhr), the very first sentence talks about intrinsic dignity by the virtue of being human. Where human rights promote the idea that dignity is inherently innate, palliative care tries to ensure that dignity is upheld even in the context of challenging illness. It has been quite interesting to look at dignity because it is so subjective. It can be enhanced or destroyed through our personal circumstances.

I think that Nouwen offers a superb quotation. I do really believe that it describes compassion perfectly—meeting the patient or the person where they are in their brokenness and illness, physically, emotionally, and spiritually, and trying to help them restore their sense of self. This really does speak to it so strongly. That said, it does not express sufficiently that compassion requires action. It is not just being there immersed in the condition of being human because you are alongside someone else who is suffering—how do we act to relieve that suffering? How do we act to ensure that because we have that sense of compassion, we seek to improve the situation?

I think a lot of people come to work in hospice because of their personal faith and how that supports them in the work that they do. Yet I still think one can be a compassionate practitioner working from a secular humanist concept because it is essentially a good thing to do. In Africa, specifically from the Xhosa Bantu language in South Africa but used more widely, we have a concept or value called *Ubuntu* which tries to explain this. *Umntu* is about the personhood of man or being; it describes a person. There is a proverb: *Umuntu ngumuntu ngabantu*—'I am a person because you are a person'. We are people together. I only can express my being and my humanity through a relationship with you or with anyone else in community. That speaks to the core values of *Ubuntu*— respect, dignity, and compassion within community. We have written a short introduction to palliative care and within that explained how the values of palliative care were reflected through *Ubuntu* and how palliative care and *Ubuntu* speak to each other. In the African context, that is very much through community.

I think that compassion is an attitude, something that can be learnt or taught, but the key message is through role modelling. The learner needs to be alongside the practitioner who demonstrates and models the attitudes of care and compassion. We know how much easier it is to transfer knowledge and develop skills but attitude is such a critical area, especially in the context of overworked health care professionals facing increasing demands. One's sense of compassion can be eroded unless you have consciously identified that this is part of how you respond to every patient, whether you find it easy to relate to them naturally or you are managing patients where their behaviour is challenging. Looking at our own programme of learning, the opportunity for practice-based role modelling is restricted partly because of cost, but more because we have few palliative care services within the country to provide the practical learning, and our students would need to take time out of their work to be able to attend, which is not usually possible. As a distance-learning programme, much of the teaching takes place online and so we develop the issue of attitudes and compassion as one example through the use of discussion groups. This can be useful.

I think it is important to understand the difference between hospice across Africa and in Europe. Speaking about South Africa in particular, hospice is mainly a nurse-led, home-based care provision based on providing care in the place where that person is. We have very few hospice facilities that have inpatient beds, and those that do are usually quite small. Our hospice in Cape Town talks about having ten beds and yet they have 900 patients. Most people will be cared for at home and often will actually die at home. We have very few doctors in hospices and in those that do, about half of them are volunteers and only 20 per cent of them have qualification in palliative care. This is a concern in ensuring that we are providing competent, in-depth palliative care. However, our greatest strength in compassionate caregiving are the home-based carers who are largely from the same community as the patient. They usually have a grade 10 education and three to four months training in palliative care, basic nursing, communication skills and counselling, and in HIV, because a lot of our patients are HIV-positive. When I spoke about this in the United States, they made the comment that legal implications prohibit volunteers carrying out any nursing function. In Africa, we would not be able to provide the care that we do without this amazing group of workers who in many cases are unpaid. We try to pay but our minimum wage is scarcely above the poverty level. These people demonstrate the most incredible compassion for the neighbours that they are helping here. That respect, dignity, and compassion all stem from this idea of *Ubuntu*.

A case exemplar

The case that really stands out for me is one of my very first patients when I was working in the hospice care. The hospice had just started, so, not wishing to overburden the voluntary GPs, nurse management asked each to be on call one night a week and do one weekend a month. It was coming up to Christmas, and there was a patient in the ward diagnosed with multiple myeloma and, because of her disease, a fractured left femur as well. I remember she was taken down to the X-ray department at the local hospital. Because of her fragile bone structure and myeloma, they fractured the opposite right humerus moving her from the trolley onto the X-ray table. So there was a woman with a fracture of her left leg and right arm—an incredible nursing challenge. This was clearly a very difficult pain problem to manage and none of us had training in palliative care. A doctor would be called at night to help with this severe pain that was almost impossible to manage. Every day there was a change in order because of the rotation of the GP cover—this doctor liked DF118 and this doctor like morphine and this doctor liked the NSAIDs. There was no continuity of care. She had to keep telling the story to different people. My heart just went out to her because she was in dreadful pain and she was not being helped. I said to my practice partner,

> You know this should not be happening. We could take over the whole running of that little ten-bed hospice. We could go in every morning and do the ward round, see this particular lady, and make sure she is getting focused pain management.

So my partner and I took over the management of medical care in the hospice who were really very grateful. Clearly the most difficult thing was the intractable pain when she was being bathed or toileted. We got her comfortable at rest—that was such an achievement. I think those are the kind of stories that really tell people why we are in palliative care—because you can make a difference to somebody whose life is unbearable because of pain. We can provide the necessary comfort and be able to interact with her family through the last weeks of her life. I think because it was one of my early patients it has really stayed with me the whole time.

Fostering sustainable compassion

In South Africa, palliative care is situated within the NGO sector. If I look at the people working in hospice today, they are doing it because they are committed, dedicated people who want to relieve suffering. That is still their aim and their goal. Many of them are not earning a market-related salary and so, partly, you might see it as a calling. I think that is another thing that seems to be linked with compassion—when the rewards or affirmation of the work that one is doing are not materially related, but is rather something that gives you a sense of making a difference in each person's life. I think that helps sustain a compassionate attitude.

The Hospice and Palliative Care Association of South Africa (HPCA) received a large grant from the United States government to integrate palliative care into our formal health care sector. We see this as an opportunity to spread the values of palliative care, including compassion and respect for our patients and colleagues, which may influence the current kind of apathy and lack of empathy that seems to be pervasive in an overburdened health system. We want to bring back compassion and caring to health care in South Africa. It may be something that we are being idealistic about; we may find we don't manage it but at least we will be trying.

Some people say it is too ambitious to bring dignity and care into a really busy public health sector. If you look at the components of Harvey Chochinov's paper that I discussed earlier, none of those take time—it is just how you behave and how you are towards your patients. Caring engenders a stronger relationship between you and the patient, so it is more rewarding and you see your job is worthwhile. I think that is so important to develop. We started this concept through our HPCA project 'Building Compassionate Communities'. We believe that the foundation of hospice care is compassion and respect for others.

We are 20 years into a democracy and the promises of democracy have not been realized by the majority of our population. We have so many disenfranchised communities. The real way to understand and to have empathy with another person is really to listen to them, and that is what we do in palliative care. That is one of the key things that make palliative care a very strong discipline. We sit and we listen, not just to the patient's symptoms, but to their experience of illness. We can do that with communities about their experience of life. It echoes the Cherokee Native American saying about not judging a man until you have walked a mile in his shoes. Karen Armstrong also speaks about that in the Compassion Charter.

So we need to take time to reach out to somebody we don't know—a colleague that we have not got to know in our work or church or child's school or community—and say, 'Why don't you tell me your story?' In South Africa, there are so many stories of people overcoming such incredible adversity and achieving such amazing things. Yet there are still people who are stuck in adversity and who need a helping hand to get out of it. We thought we could publish those stories, with the persons' permission, on e-hospice, or even publish them on the Compassion Charter website and just see where this leads. Just the telling of the story is therapeutic. We may find that builds understanding between communities. South Africa has got such a high rate of violence and crime that I think it is also rooted in the feeling of being disenchanted. We will never solve all the problems of the world in this way, but just one step at a time will help one person, even a little bit.

Of course, this is not a new concept. Allan Kellehear from Australia has written extensively on this, as has Karen Armstrong with her push for the

Compassion Charter. As well, there are many compassionate care programmes around the world, including Suresh Kumar's in Kerala. Then there is the wonderful writing from those such as Archbishop Desmond Tutu and the Dalai Lama. I remember in a HPCA blog from October 2011, acknowledging the 80th birthday of Desmond Tutu, I wrote:

Archbishop Tutu and the Dalai Lama are both inspirational leaders who speak of the importance of compassion. Archbishop Tutu writes that 'I have consciously sought during my life to emulate my mother, whom our family knew as a gentle comforter of the afflicted' (Tutu & Allen 2010: vi). The Dalai Lama reflects upon 'what binds us all together, the essential elements of our common humanity and the compassion it calls for' (Dalai Lama & Stril-Rever 2010: 7).

That to me feels like a watershed. It is time for our communities to say we have had enough of the war and terror. Surely the way to change the war and terror is to understand the roots of where it comes from and to build those bridges.

Commentary

Chokyi Nyima Rinpoche and David Shima (2006) describe the vow a *bodhisattva* takes to care for all sentient beings as *bodhichitta*—'enlightened resolve'. The resolve requires both effort and bravery because the person taking this resolve is saying that they want to do better at being compassionate towards all sentient beings no matter how long it takes or what obstacles are put in the way. The resolve requires the seeker to pay attention to six virtues, all of which speak to the way in which we practice palliative and end-of-life care and, presumably, health care in general. Briefly, these pertain to being generous (doing whatever is necessary to provide comfort), being conscientious (doing the right thing immediately), tolerance, perseverance (sometimes called joyous diligence!), pure concentration (paying attention), and intelligence. The last is most important of all since it underpins all the other virtues of enlightened resolve. Intelligence is about wisdom and open-mindedness to both process and outcome.

The desire to bring compassionate communities to the people of South Africa as expressed here by Liz Gwyther attest to the ideal of enlightened resolve. There is an energy evoked by the desire to take action, the desire to bring about change for the good of all. Although the practice of compassionate palliative and end-of-life care by its nature focuses on the relationship between the patient, family, and clinician, the wider context of changing society is also important. The richness of *Ubuntu* speaks not only to African society but offers important messages to us all. The blessing of *Ubuntu* as a foundation for how society works at the community level means, hopefully, that what Liz Gwyther seeks in a compassionate South African society will awaken readily (and the lessons learnt will be of use to) the global palliative care community. The Desmond Tutu Peace Foundation (http://www.tutufoundation-usa.org) organized an inter-spiritual breakfast in 2008 called 'Seeds of Compassion', which presented a dialogue on the topic between the archbishop and the Dalai Lama. Desmond Tutu remarks that compassion requires that 'we be gentle with ourselves, so we can be gentle with others.' The case exemplar of a patient with myeloma is certainly indicative of the gentleness of approach that is often needed in being able to manage their fragility, whether that be physical, psychological, social, or spiritual. Being open to the virtues which frame 'enlightened resolve' may enhance the gentle nature of the compassionate response.

Reflections for practice

◆ Consider where the importance of being gentle was a catalyst for change in your professional practice? Why was that necessary? Why did it work?

◆ Where in your work have you seen concepts allied to *Ubuntu* practised? What enabled those concepts to be valued?

◆ What is needed in palliative and end-of-life care practice today to ensure that the values of *Ubuntu* are not lost to the global development of clinical practice?

Further reading

Chochinov H (2007) Dignity and the essence of medicine: the A, B, C, and D of dignity conserving care. British Medical Journal, **335**, 184–187.

Kellehear A (2013) Compassionate communities: end-of-life care as everyone's responsibility. QJM: An International Journal of Medicine, **106**(12), 1071–1075.

Dalai Lama, Stril-Rever S (2010) My spiritual journey. New York: HarperCollins.

Radbruch L, deLima L, Lohmann D, Gwyther E, Payne S (2013) The Prague Charter: urging governments to relieve suffering and ensure the right to palliative care. Palliative Medicine, **27**(2), 101–102.

Rinpoche CN, Shima D (2006) Medicine and compassion: a Tibetan lama's guidance for caregivers. Somerville, MA: Wisdom Publications.

Seeds of Compassion (2008) The Desmond Tutu Peace Foundation. http://www.tutufoundation-usa.org

Tutu D, Allen J (2010) God is not a Christian: speaking truth in times of crisis. London: Rider.

Tutu D, Tutu M (2014) The book of forgiving: the fourfold path for healing ourselves and our world. New York: HarperCollins.

Chapter 14

Jo Hockley—Spirit

Jo Hockley trained as a nurse at St Bartholomew's Hospital, London, in the early 1970s and has worked in specialist palliative care for over 30 years, most recently as nurse consultant at St Christopher's Hospice in London. She has had a passion for disseminating palliative care knowledge within generalist settings. During her career she has set up two hospital-based palliative care teams (St Bartholomew's Hospital, London, and Western General Hospital, Edinburgh) and more recently a care home project team serving over 100 care homes at St Christopher's Hospice, based on results from her PhD. Jo has published widely both on the strategic development of hospital-based palliative care teams and palliative care for older people in care homes. She has recently been awarded an OBE for her contributions to palliative care nursing.

Foundations in palliative and end-of-life care

I don't come from a nursing family and I think what motivated me to come into nursing then motivated me to come into hospice care. One of the reasons I came into nursing was to help people who were suffering, not necessarily to get better, but to help them in their suffering. As a Christian, I was motivated to do something more than office work. I did my training at Barts (St. Bartholomew's Hospital) for four years. I then went off to be a midwife and went to Africa to work voluntarily with a missionary society for nine months. I came back to the UK thinking of going back into oncology. However, my brother had worked at St Christopher's Hospice for a month as part of his theological training, and he said, 'Why don't you go and work at St Christopher's?' My immediate thought was, 'This is crazy, my work is about birth.' However, I decided to 'check out' St Christopher's and arranged to meet the matron (director of nursing).

As I walked into the hospice I immediately noticed the incredibly professional yet humane care they were giving in a very natural way. I just thought this is where I want to go and work. I only planned to work there for six months, but within three months they asked me to apply for a ward sister's job. I stayed as a ward sister for four years. Then I thought the world needs to hear about the hospice movement. This was around 1982, and that is really what formulated my passion for trying to disseminate hospice principles into the generalist setting.

I was appointed as a clinical nurse specialist (CNS) in palliative care back at Barts to initially undertake some research and then set up one of the first hospital-based palliative care teams in London.

After nine years it was time for a change. I didn't want to go into full-time management or education, and yet I realized, at the age of 40, I needed to go to university and do a master's if I wanted to stay as a CNS. I went to Edinburgh for a year to do that and took the time out and funded myself. Towards the end of that year, I was being encouraged to come back to St Christopher's and apply for the director of nursing post but, in fact, I stayed in Scotland and set up a second hospital-based palliative care team. I have been fortunate in my career as I feel as if opportunities have presented themselves to me without too much effort on my part! A colleague mentioned that there was an advert to do a PhD looking at end-of-life care in care homes. For the past 12 years that has been my focus.

Looking at end-of-life care for very old people in care homes has taught me even more about dying than when I was in specialist palliative care. I think that there is greater complexity within the hospice movement now than there was in the late 70s and early 80s when I was there. Much of the work in hospices has been with people dying in midlife from cancer, and their families—the trauma of grief in young children. With frail older people in care homes it is different. Yes, pain is a problem, but generally it is about much more than simply prescribing analgesia. It is more about encouraging staff to see dying as the end of a long life lived rather than failure of care. There are not so many people in care homes dying from cancer. Residents in care homes often have a number of diseases—one of which may be cancer, but more often is dementia, circulatory disease, or heart disease. I have really had to readjust my thinking from 'Yes, people need morphine in order to die well.' Frail older people can die very well with very little medication and that has been a huge learning curve for me. I think there is a danger of imposing hospice principles established around cancer on the frail older people dying in care homes. I think it is much more about collaboration, learning about the difference in frail older people, and working together. I used to think 'I know how to care for people at the end of life', but I have learnt so much from nurses/carers in nursing homes. The four years I did at St Christopher's Hospice was just a starting block for me. Many times I think frail older people know they are going to die; I think there may be something biological that helps older people to be more accepting that their life has come to a natural end, and that is a very different thing for people dying in midlife from cancer.

I always thought that grief in nursing homes wasn't necessarily such an issue as in hospices. My dad died from a cancer when I was 25. It was shocking and I can remember at the time thinking, 'I hope not too many other people have to go through this.' However, I had the whole of my life before me and that was able to distract me from the grief. Prior to my mother's death two years ago, aged ninety-nine and a half, I was thinking, 'Mum has had a good life; she is ready to go.' She died reasonably quickly. But I was surprised by the grief I felt. The difference between my father's death and my mother's death was that my mother had been around for 63 years of my life, and there was that greater tearing apart. I think it would be interesting to look at grief in care homes, especially for those bereaved people who are single, who have had a lot of involvement with their father or their mother. At present little attention is given to grief in care homes.

The compassionate practitioner

I remember being very aware of compassionate care while working at St Christopher's Hospice. We had such good role models. I saw a humanity there that enabled me to be human. I was able to be me. It was about taking off that professional mask that we tend to wrap ourselves in, especially the training that we had back in the 70s. There was this 'stiff upper lip'; you don't sit on the bed, etc. In many ways that was such a barrier. I still gave compassionate care but perhaps didn't recognize it for what it was. I remember once when working in the oncology ward, one patient called me over just as I was going off duty and said, 'Staff Nurse Hockley, there is something different about you, what is it?' I should have stayed and asked her whether she could explain further but I wanted to get off duty and was also embarrassed! So, I believe it was there.

For me, being compassionate is being human. Everyone is busy but it is about using time well with patients and families. You can have an incredibly compassionate conversation but it does not necessarily need to be half an hour long. It is more than conversation; it is about your attitude, obviously to people, but also about how one does all one's work. I think compassion is also about earning respect from patients and families so that they can trust you, and then they feel they can open up to you. I think it is about spirituality. It is about an awakening within us to be compassionate.

I don't think people start out necessarily at 20 being full of compassion but it can grow. I would say that I had a level of compassion when I came into nursing but as I have grown older I have become more passionate as a person. I am a much more compassionate person now at a deeper level. It is something that grows. I came into nursing to help people. I can remember being very happy as a midwife but I found my raison d'être caring for people at the end of life. It has been a surprise to me, but it is an area of care that has held me. Compassion is also about acknowledging our mistakes. It is about being aware of ourselves and then trying to be a better person in our work, and trying to connect—not just do a job. I do fear that because of the busyness of work in our current health care we will revert again back to the task-orientated approach.

Compassion was integral to my nurse training. Although it was not called that then—it was about caring. It sort of oozed from the bricks and mortar at Barts. Barts was founded in 1123 by monks at the monastery of St Bartholomew the Great. So it always had that underpinning of care from a spiritual sense. It was integral to how we did nursing. I went into nursing at a slightly older age and admit I hadn't a clue. My first ward sister appeared very strict and aloof. Luckily the ward closed for decoration and I went up to another ward where the ward sister was an incredibly compassionate role model. I suppose I felt valued. She valued me and I think that is an important part of compassion. People can have compassion within them but unless they feel valued it is sometimes difficult for the compassionate person to emerge.

Nowadays we *talk* a lot about spiritual care and holistic care, but to be honest with you, sometimes I don't see it being carried out. I believe one of problems in the last 20 years has been the emphasis on targets and systems rather than valuing the person doing the work. I think compassion can get squashed out when pressures are too great. If people don't feel valued it is very difficult for them to keep that compassion topped up for patients and families. One of the ways of not valuing staff for what they do is to cut their numbers. We need to bring a greater humanity into the system.

For my PhD I looked at Habermas and his systems theory: the theory of communicative action. He talks about the importance of systems being of *equal* importance to that of the lifeworld (i.e. people) and not people as part of a subsystem of the system. I see people being part of a subsystem sometimes! I think what was so valuable about the hospice movement in the 70s and 80s was that system worked well because staff were valued for what they gave, and they gave really great compassionate end-of-life care. One of those things which I see being eroded is 'being with' someone who is dying. That was such a core, fundamental aspect of end-of-life care, you sat with somebody, and it was something I had to learn.

I can remember when I was first in charge of a late shift at St Christopher's. I had been there about two months, and matron did a ward round of all the patients before she went home at six o'clock. I had just finished the six o'clock drugs and she said to me, 'Staff Nurse Hockley, did you realize that the lady in Room 7 is dying?' I had not recognized it. Here was I, an oncology nurse, and I had not recognized dying. She said, 'If you just draw up a little diamorphine and hyoscine, I will go and sit with her.' So I drew it up, went into the room, and gave the injection. She was sitting next to the patient, and as I went to walk out of the room, Matron said, 'No, just come and sit, the girls can manage the rest of the patients, your priority is here.' We sat together for about 40 minutes during which time the lady breathed her last breath. Matron was role modelling the importance of 'being with' the dying and the importance of valuing that time. There is a huge danger that if we are not careful we are going to lose the compassion around end-of-life care.

The palliative care physician Michael Kearney talks about the danger of just being 'symptomatologists' (Kearney 1992). I think we are seeing that doctors and nurses are interested in symptom control because it is a tangible thing, where 'being with' the dying is more difficult. However, it is what underpinned the hospice movement. Sitting with someone dying, we feel frail ourselves; we feel vulnerable with the patient. It is important to be able to feel vulnerable, to be able to identify with the patients and their families; it reveals our humanity. If we never feel vulnerable we are going to be incredibly hard and it will be difficult then to allow compassion to grow.

I think we can teach compassion but it must also be role modelled. In education I think you can be seen to be compassionate about how you share case studies and how you lecture. I think you can be seen to be compassionate about how you listen to someone who is trying to ask you a question who is not particularly articulate—to take time to try to help them explain what it is they want to say in front of the rest of the class. You can role model compassion whether you are in the education room or whether you are in the clinical situation. I do think it is something we can nurture in people.

A case exemplar

One situation stands out above all the others! At the time, I was a clinical nurse specialist on the palliative care team. I had been asked to visit this Scottish woman in one of the wards. She had been married but her husband walked out of the marriage and left her with their six-month little boy. She travelled to London to get work. Thirty years later, she was diagnosed with cancer of the cervix. She had it treated radically with radiotherapy but ten years later returned with a second primary as a result of the initial radiotherapy. This was when I was asked to see her.

She could have had radical surgery and further chemotherapy but she refused any further treatment outright. She said to me she was an agnostic and the idea was for our team to help persuade her to go to the local hospice. But she totally refused. The consultant kindly allowed her to stay in the surgical ward, which would not happen nowadays. I therefore got to know her well over two and a half months as we tried to support her and control her symptoms. She got angry when she saw other people on the ward die and she was 'allowed to suffer'. On one occasion she had asked me to give her euthanasia. I felt awkward. She was clearly very ill—and I believed she wanted to die. She was being nursed on a special bed because she was so thin, in a long, old-fashioned, Nightingale-type ward. We had her pain and other symptoms well controlled but there was no way I could commit euthanasia—anyway, it is not legalized in the UK. Elizabeth was very determined that she just wanted to die, but she could not die.

She fascinated me as a person. I knew she would never have a priest come to see her—she was very angry with them as well! However, I felt there was a very deep emotional or spiritual need. I was not sure what it was. We sat as nurses on the ward and discussed it and I said, 'You see whether you can help her emotionally—perhaps there is a tie with her son that is making her hold on to this life, and I will see if I can do anything on the spiritual side.' At least a month went by and I did not have the courage to address it. It requires one to step out of their comfort zone sometimes when we are giving compassionate care.

I was about to go on holiday for a second time and thought, I must try to address this issue. I was sitting by her the day before I went on holiday. If anybody else had been there I would have said they said it, but clearly I did! I asked her, 'Elizabeth, before I go would you like me to pray for you?' And much to my surprise, she said 'Yes'! This all going on in the middle of visiting hours, on a Wednesday afternoon with all the visitors around various people's beds. I did not want to pull the curtains around the bed in case people thought something was up and started listening in to our conversation. So I said to Elizabeth, 'You close your eyes, and I will pray for you.' I can remember to this day the words I said. I said, 'Father, Elizabeth cannot understand how there can be a God of love because of the disappointments she has had in her life. I just pray that you will show her your love in Jesus on the cross', at which point I felt I was standing on hallowed ground! My hands were shaking.

I opened my eyes to see that Elizabeth was Cheyne-Stokes breathing. It was terrifying! All I can remember thinking was, 'Not only have you been praying for a patient, Jo' (something that was not strictly allowed), 'but she is now going to die without the curtains round the bed!' I sat and waited. It was probably only about two to three minutes, but it felt like ten minutes, when suddenly she opened her eyes, turned to me, and said, 'Jo, thank you *so* much.' Unfortunately I did not have the presence of mind at the time to ask what was going on for Elizabeth. She clearly had had an out-of-body experience. Instead I just said, 'Oh well, Elizabeth, I will come and see you first thing in the morning before I go on holiday.' The next day, just as I was finishing chatting to her, she said, 'Jo, before you go, would you pray for me like you did yesterday?' So I did—it was just a normal little prayer, nothing like the day before—and I left.

A week later I came back from holiday to find out that the very day I had left to go on holiday, Elizabeth had asked someone to read from the Bible This person didn't know what to read but turned to Psalm 23 thinking that was what people found comfort in. As she began reading the psalm she struggled with verse 5—'Though I walk through the valley of the shadow of death, I will fear no evil'—this must have been such a comfort to Elizabeth but scary for the nurse to say aloud as one does not talk about death and dying in an acute hospital ward. Anyway, the next day she asked somebody else to read from the Bible, and that night she died in her sleep. The following day, a Roman Catholic nurse came in having not been around. She knew Elizabeth had died as she had dreamt about her the previous night—and told the nurses about the dream: Elizabeth was sitting out of bed, smiling, and all dressed in white. Elizabeth had not been out of bed in ten weeks.

For me, it was a profound example of compassionate care as spiritual healing. I learnt a lot about going that extra mile with Elizabeth and giving real holistic care, but it had involved risk. There were issues that she had needed to resolve within herself; I wasn't privy to what those issues were. However, I needed to step out of my comfort zone to give what I believed was compassionate, holistic care. Whatever happened, Elizabeth gained peace and it was a privilege to be the vehicle for that.

I think the Henri Nouwen definition speaks to that. I was not comfortable going where I went with her. These days it is even harder to take risks because of the fear of legal repercussions. I think that can undermine holistic care. When I think back over this situation, I still would have done it today, but then I don't mind risk. If she had said, 'No, I do not want you to pray for me', well then, obviously, I would not have prayed for her. However, it felt very risky and took me a number of weeks before I addressed her request for euthanasia through compassionate spiritual care. It taught me that it is OK to ask someone if they want you to pray for them, without imposing one's faith on people. It is the same as offering a hug or putting an arm around someone. It is about taking that risk. Compassion really asks us to go the extra mile.

Fostering sustainable compassion

We are all responsible for this. Caring compassionately over many years for people who are dying and their families can demoralize some people. People need to feel valued for the work they do—but there is huge pressure on resources, which sometimes makes this difficult. However, it is not just about resources. When I was first at St Christopher's, Dame Cicely Saunders would eat at the same table as us. That was a profound thing for me. Nowadays we are much more in our own silos. The emphasis on systems and targets immediately devalues people.

When I first worked at St Christopher's, we were allowed four mental health days. If you really felt it was all getting to you, you could take time for yourself to recharge your batteries. I can't say that I ever took any but it is very unlikely that one is given them these days. Not everyone is the same and we must remember this—we are all unique with different gifts and ways of using them, but we all need to feel valued to bring out the best in us. Some people can take a huge amount of pressure; others cannot. I think we do need to foster compassion within the hospice movement and now is a very critical time with second and third generations. Compassion and sitting with the dying and opening up conversations with the dying are difficult things to do—but it is what Dame Cicely did best. It was her compassion for the original Polish gentleman who had no family, in a different country, dying of cancer. Her heart went out to him.

Another way people felt valued when working at St Christopher's was that every month Dame Cicely and one or two other doctors would sit down at a ward meeting to talk over issues that staff had raised. At such a meeting I was rather shocked when the ward sister said to me, 'Staff Nurse Hockley, we were chatting earlier this week about a lady you felt was having too much sedation and you were concerned about euthanasia. Do want to share your thoughts?' At the time I was surprised that my comment had been picked up but there was a real concern to discuss these really important issues that young nurses and young doctors raised when they came into specialist palliative care. There was an openness and a valuing of people's opinions. We need to be careful that the innate compassion within us does not get squashed. I know many organizations where people say, 'Jo, I don't feel valued here, you know, nobody mentions me by my name.' So people leave and there is a high turnover and it's a downward spiral.

One thing that sparks my interest is *mindfulness*. Loads of people are talking about mindfulness. I think mindfulness is a bit like compassion but I don't think it quite has the same depth as I understand compassion—'come-with-passion'. I think we have to have something stirring within us to make us passionate enough about it, to be able to be a compassionate practitioner. Compassion has to come alight somehow; one has to demonstrate compassion—then professionals need to be willing to allow it to stay alight within themselves.

Commentary

Jo Hockley is one of a number of contributors to this book who consider that their faith brought them to the field of health care and then into palliative and end-of-life care. In reading her own letters, it is important to remember how important the Christian faith was to Cicely Saunders in her thinking about the development of palliative and hospice care and her desire to blend medical and spiritual aspects of care, which came to mean the whole-person approach which embodies the practice today (Clark 2002). Jo Hockley also speaks to the interchangeable description of hospice and palliative care which may be relatively Anglo-centric in its thinking and different to the way in which it is perceived in other parts of the world. Further, her concerns regarding the bureaucratization of health care are reminiscent of early critique by Bradshaw (1996) about the abandonment of Christian 'charism' from health care institutions. From the case study, that faith and belief in a deeper spiritual context governing our lives enabled a transformative process to ease the suffering of Elizabeth. The Dominican author Michael Dodds wrote that the question of where is God in the midst of human suffering 'plumbs the depths of our theology but also touches the heart of our human experience' (p. 330).

As palliative care practitioners, we are particularly exposed to the suffering of others, to their losses, disappointments, and fears as well as, hopefully, some of the joys in their lives. Christina Feldman (2005) would argue that we are not expected to endure someone else's suffering but rather to 'open your heart to embrace the realities of life' (p. 52). In the face of suffering, the compassionate response of the practitioner enables the heart to remain open to possibility and transformation. Another important issue raised here is the acceptance of dying. Camilla Zimmerman (2012) explored the idea of acceptance of death as the sociological antithesis of death denial and argued that palliative care extols a good death as one in which the patient has accepted the inevitable and therefore is accessible to the care interventions provided. Only if death is accepted can it be managed within the health care system. However, it is not unknown in palliative and end-of-life care that the patient has accepted the reality of dying but death does not occur (as in the case of Elizabeth). Then compassion requires the wisdom to question every aspect of our practice to see how we can be present for those who suffer when we may feel at the limit of clinical power.

Reflections for practice

+ Do you consider having a religious faith or spiritual practice important in the delivery of compassionate care?
+ In the case of Elizabeth, how would you respond to her anger at being unable to die?
+ What are your views on the idea that death needs to be accepted in order for it to be well-managed?

Further reading

Bradshaw A (1996) The spiritual dimension of hospice: the secularization of an ideal. Social Science & Medicine, **43**, 409–419.

Clark D (2002) Cicely Saunders: founder of the hospice movement. Selected letters, 1959–1999. Oxford: Oxford University Press.

Dodds M (1991) Thomas Aquinas, human suffering and the unchanging God of love. Theological Studies, **52**, 330–344.

Feldman C (2005) Compassion: listening to the cries of the world. Berkeley, CA: Rodmell.

Habermas J (1987) Theory of communicative action. Vol. II: Lifeworld and system: a critique of functionalist reason (transl. T McCarthy). Cambridge: Polity Press.

Kearney M (1992) Palliative medicine—just another specialty? Palliative Medicine, 6(1), 39–46.

Zimmerman C (2012) Acceptance of dying: a discourse analysis of palliative care literature. Social Science & Medicine, **75(1)**, 217–224.

Chapter 15

Peter Hudson—Vulnerability

Professor Peter Hudson is a registered nurse with more than 25 years' experience in palliative care practice, education, and research. He is a board member of Palliative Care Australia and was a director of the board of the International Association for Hospice and Palliative Care for six years. Peter is co-founder and chair of the International Palliative Care Family Carer Research Collaboration (http://www.ipcfrc.centreforpallcare.org), which operates under the auspices of the European Association of Palliative Care (EAPC), and was co-leader of an EAPC task force aimed at enhancing support provided to family carers.

Peter is director of the Centre for Palliative Care (St Vincent's Hospital and Collaborative Centre of the University of Melbourne, Australia), honorary professor at the University of Melbourne, and professor of palliative care at Queen's University, Belfast (UK). The Centre for Palliative Care (http://www.centreforpallcare.org) has a statewide role in palliative care education and research in Victoria. It focuses on the development of evidence-based practice through research and education, with networks and collaborative projects extending nationally and internationally. Peter's role is to oversee the development of research programmes covering palliative care service delivery, psychosocial support, and symptom management. He has a particular interest in developing and evaluating strategies to improve the psychosocial support for families affected by advanced disease.

He has published more than 50 international peer-reviewed journal articles as the lead author. In 2009, he co-edited a book (published by Oxford University Press) focusing on ways to improve the evidence-based support to family carers of patients diagnosed with life-threatening illness. Peter has received several awards including a postdoctoral research award (Nurses' Board of Victoria); presentation award from the Third Research Forum of the European Association for Palliative Care, and the premiers' award for evidence-based practice. He is affiliated with more than 15 professional national and international organizations in palliative care, nursing, and other health-related fields.

He also established and coordinates the multidisciplinary graduate certificate in palliative care (via the University of Melbourne), aimed at preparing health care professionals for specialist palliative care provision. He oversees several other training initiatives including professional development programmes and discipline-specific specialist education.

Foundations in palliative and end-of-life care

I trained in Australia and my nursing career postgraduation was very much focused on intensive care and cardiothoracics. I realized that much of my time in intensive care was not involved in conversing with patients and families. Patients were typically intubated and family visits were infrequent, particularly if I was on night duty. I felt that I was more of a technician and less of a nurse. My wife, who was working at the Royal Marsden Hospital, actually suggested that I try community nursing, and so I was exposed to my first palliative care patient through interaction with McMillan Nursing. We were in London at that time and that is where my appetite for palliative care was born. I did some Marie Curie night-sitting in London and returned back to Melbourne, Australia. I was hooked. Something grabbed me about looking after dying patients and families. I felt I had the opportunity to be a nurse again and for me that was a chance to converse with patients and families; to take time to listen to them and provide holistic care. I found there were too many barriers to those areas in the acute setting at the time.

I furthered my clinical nursing career in palliative care and in due course became a coordinator of a palliative care home-based programme. I thoroughly enjoyed my clinical work; however, I was constantly concerned about the lack of evidence that underpinned much of the palliative care practice at the time in the early to mid-90s. I had a lot of questions that seemed unanswered. I suppose I had a thirst for research and that led me to undertake a PhD in the area of family caregiver support; I undertook a psycho-educational intervention with a randomized control trial which focused on trying to better prepare family members for the role of looking after someone who is dying at home. My desire for research and training grew and further opportunities came up professionally to take a position at the Centre for Palliative Care at Melbourne University, which is where I am now. The centre is a multidisciplinary academic unit based at St Vincent's Hospital, recognized as a collaborative centre at the University of Melbourne. We have a statewide remit, focusing on three areas of research in palliative care: psychosocial support for patients and families, health service evaluation models of palliative care provision, and clinical drug trials. We are also involved in a number of multidisciplinary and uni-disciplinary palliative care training initiatives.

My passion is still to answer some of the key questions in palliative care and improve the skill set of multiprofessional health care providers so that they can support patients and families at end of life in a much more appropriate way. In Australia, as in many other parts of the world, most of the people with life-threatening, advanced, incurable disease will be looked after outside specialist care. Most of our health care workforce come out of their undergraduate training with virtually no palliative care formal training whatsoever. No matter where they end up working, they will all be required to look after a dying patient and family at some stage.

The compassionate practitioner

For me I think it is about acknowledging somebody's suffering and that acknowledgement evoking some desire in me to try to address that, which may not always be possible. I think the Nouwen definition is pertinent. I realize the definition comes from a Christian perspective but I don't think that faith is in any way a prerequisite for palliative care. I have worked with many colleagues from secular backgrounds and have seen very explicit examples of compassion. I don't think it is imperative.

I must admit in our training programmes we don't formally teach compassion. I have never been on the receiving end of a lecture or tutorial on how to be more compassionate, but I think it should be possible, albeit indirectly. Some of the tenets of communication training are relevant and there are some excellent frameworks with regard to communication at the end of life. There might be some lessons learnt here pertinent to teaching compassion to health care professionals. From the outset, we try right to unpack what palliative care is and I think by exploring explicitly some of the standards and principles of palliative care, we hopefully change attitudes for those people who perhaps thought that palliative care was a little bit soft, or something different. We are able to articulate what palliative care is, what the essence of palliative care is, and through examples demonstrate how compassionate palliative care can make a difference. Perhaps we do it less explicitly than we should. Role modelling is helpful as I think the face-to-face exposure and a mentorship approach is most desirable, but I would not necessarily conclude that it is the only successful way. Case studies could also work.

When I first studied palliative care, we studied the birth of the modern hospice movement and several references to Cicely Saunders which led you to question your attitudes. She was an obvious role model. When you go through her background and some of the examples of compassion that she undertook, you can just see the audience change—particularly those people who did not know who she was and what she achieved. Many people in the generalist health care workforce would not know who Cicely Saunders is. Exposing people to that foundation actually has benefit in itself.

I think there are other examples of compassion, not limited to verbalizing support for somebody. I am thinking about compassion in the context of somebody who is unconscious or cognitively impaired, or where people are very close to death. It is not uncommon for health care professionals, particularly those trained in palliative care, to talk to the patient as they have been approaching the last hours of their lives and to care compassionately for the body after death in a very respectful way. So, it is more than being able to engage in conversation and express concern.

These same principles apply when you are working with the carer. It is acknowledging somebody's difficulty, distress, suffering, and having clear expectations of what palliative care can offer on both sides. A lot of patients and families are not really clear what palliative care can and can't do. We need to be explicit that palliative care is trying to help support the family as best we can in whatever way we can, acknowledging the difficulty of the situation.

The other thing that is common in palliative care is the willingness to go the extra mile. I think we may not always verbalize that but hopefully that is actioned and is seen in feedback that we will often get from patients and family—the service was willing to do a lot more than the other areas of health care that they had experienced. So I think the compassion we have for patients extends quite easily to families. I don't see any major distinction.

I was also thinking about what happens when you expect staff to be compassionate and that does not happen or is hard to apply. I think there are different ways of seeing compassion in palliative care; it occurs at a number of different levels by default: we think of a health care professional displaying compassion for a patient. In my experience, I have also witnessed patients showing compassion to me. I remember looking after a woman who had an awful fungating perineal wound which required multiple daily dressings, dreadful odour and painful. I recall doing her dressing and she could see that I was uncomfortable and she said, 'It is OK, Peter. I am not in pain, it is alright, you can keep going with the dressing, you are not hurting me.' I think there have been other examples of that ilk, where I would see the patient recognizing that I am struggling a little bit. I also think of examples of families showing compassion for the health care team, as well as their relative. I think there are many different ways of actually thinking about compassion.

A case exemplar

The one that sticks out for me is the compassion that was shown to a serial paedophile by the palliative care team. He was an incarcerated serial offender. It is not uncommon for the team to care for prisoners because the hospital we are linked to has a prison ward. Referrals come through the consultancy service.

The standard approach is we never discuss the crime. Sometimes that is exposed through discussion in the unit and in this case it was in the public domain, but it is not something that is sought by the palliative care team. We are more interested in a holistic assessment rather than trying to discern what crime has or hasn't been committed. That is never discussed. I think if people do know what crime was committed, it may lead to some internal struggle. However, for the most part there is not much fuss made about it—this is what we do. Our core work is to help people and alleviate their suffering whether it be physical, psychological, social, or spiritual. That is why we exist.

From what I have seen within the team, compassion is there irrespective of the background story. I was extremely impressed by the way in which the team provided care to this man in a very non-judgemental way. You could see how people worked collectively to determine best care. Care was provided like it would have been to anybody else. There was critical attention to symptom management and psychosocial support. The care was not compromised at all because this person had committed an awful crime. I think it helped that this was a fairly mature team and all members had training in specialist palliative care provision so they operated in a non-judgemental way with the end gain, the relief of suffering. I think supervision helps. It is pretty commonplace in psychiatry and psycho-oncology where it seems to work pretty well, certainly in Australia. The palliative care consultants would spend a lot of time in terms of nurturing staff with opportunities for feedback. It may not be as formalized as within psychiatry and psychology but nonetheless it occurs. In nursing I would describe it as haphazard and non-structured. I am not saying there is not support there but it lacks structure and is far from ideal. I think it is fairly self-evident in social work.

Literature around compassion would often talk about the need to reach out to people who are perhaps more vulnerable or in some way disenfranchised or marginalized in society. They often cite populations in prison as an example of that. I wonder if you almost need to have greater compassion in that sense because of the nature of the situation that the patient finds himself in. I have been mulling this over and I wonder if you need to readjust your compassionate response in certain circumstances. I think it helps where the focus of the organization is on caring for minority groups. We have an outreach service to the homeless and also a comprehensive programme for drug users, so it is core to the values of the organization that people are treated equally. Compassion is actually one of those values and the organization does try to action their values rather than having them sitting on the website. This case is a very good example of how they action that.

Fostering sustainable compassion

I am not sure if there is a single word to describe a lack of compassion, but I think it is sometimes about suboptimal care coordination. I do a weekly session with the clinical consult team at the facility that I am involved with and what I witness is just the level of acuity and complex needs of the patients and families. I think the services that refer to the palliative care consultancy service may struggle with managing complexity of the patient and their family. This is where palliative care can actually make a difference. The things that are elementary to palliative care can be quite difficult for other services and health care professionals—conversations about goals of care, recognizing dying, and family support—they are often very difficult for those units who do not have the training in palliative care. I would not label them as lacking in compassion, but they may lack the skills and training resources to comprehensively manage what are very difficult and complex situations.

Sometimes in palliative care we get surprised by people being offered certain treatments and interventions which, on reflection, we wish had not been offered; focus could have been more on quality of life, particularly where it seems that the intervention is futile. I do believe that in those situations where an intervention seems inappropriate, the intention of the health care professional was good, if somewhat misguided. I would see they are trying to support the patient as best they can. If they had received better training, more exposure to alternative options, then perhaps their practice might change.

I do worry about the future of palliative care. In Australia, there is an ongoing, uphill battle to have palliative care recognized and appropriately resourced, despite all the facts that we now have in terms of inequity of access and its benefits when access is possible. I think for those lucky enough to receive specialist palliative care support, compassion is a large part of that. However, over 50 per cent of people in Australia do not have access to specialist palliative care, so I worry that they are not getting the compassionate care that they have a right to receive. I also question the quality of care provided in residential age care facilities, nursing homes—these places that are becoming modern hospices. End-of-life care in some centres is very good; however, in many others it is not. We have many problems associated with trying influence that in a political way; there are a couple of national initiatives trying to address that around advance care planning and resources for those staff working in age care facilities to be able to access advice. Hopefully, the landscape may change a little, but I do worry about care in those areas.

I think we need a number of change initiatives, certainly at policy level, but absolutely in training. I mean, if somebody is working in paediatric care in this country, they would expect you to have formal training to look after newborn babies. That is not happening at end of life in this country, and to me that is illogical and very unfair for many people who are receiving suboptimal care.

As I mentioned earlier, most Australian health care professionals will start practising without any training in palliative care whatsoever. We can't expect them to provide optimal quality end-of-life care if they have not received training on how to do that. I would hope that most people who go into health care work usually do so because they want to help people, and the desire to care compassionately is instilled in all the health care professionals. There is very little evidence of palliative care in undergraduate curricula although there is an Australian national initiative underway to try to embed palliative care throughout all the relevant health care disciplines' undergraduate curricula called PCC4U (http://www.pcc4u.org). That is hopefully going to have a major influence, but as is the case in many countries, there is limited space for content within curricula. It is a matter of trying to make palliative care a priority and to influence university curriculum desires in such a way that they can ensure that there is core palliative care content included in all their undergraduate programmes in health care. That is the aim.

I feel people who should be able to avail themselves of palliative care are missing out. There is all sorts of discussion, dialogue, and debate about who is worthy of specialist care and who is not. At the moment, there is no systematic way of triaging patients as to whether or not they would benefit from a referral to palliative care, so we do not know what we can offer and to whom. The monitoring is suboptimal and patient and family needs change from day to day. Assumptions are often based on insufficient assessment which fails to respond to rapid change in the patient's condition. General health care professionals and family members involved in that care need to be able to pick up on some of those signs, and know how to get additional support by way of specialist palliative care.

I think at the moment there is not a consumer-driven agenda for enhancing palliative care. Palliative care in Australia is publicly funded and some of the services survive on charitable donations, but it is not the expectation. It is not a situation like in the UK, for example, where the community are seemingly a bit more aware of what hospice and palliative care is. That is not the case in Australia. Some of my friends do not know what it is that I do. I have been doing this for almost 30 years, and they think what I do is a bit peculiar but they don't really understand it; they find it difficult to fathom that there would be some benefit from researching in palliative care. The common suggestion is people are approaching their death, so what else can you do?

There are many misconceptions about palliative care in Australia. Death is pretty much hidden in our country at the moment. Most family members have not looked after a dying person before. They have not seen a dead body before. Although I am probably generalizing, there is a public perception that death is always horrible, painful, and distressing, and although it can be, it is also possible that the lead-up to death is not painful. I have heard family describe how he went so peacefully; it was a beautiful death; his time came; he was well supported; he was comfortable. We don't hear enough about these stories. We hear about the negative aspects of death and dying and that is fuelling the euthanasia debate in this country and many others.

A lot more needs to be done to address some of those misconceptions. I think it would be advantageous if there was a stronger consumer voice to try help with a palliative care agenda so that there can be a sustained marketing communications plan around demystifying what palliative care is. I suppose what we are striving for is better palliative care service, and I think we are pushing for that with our government to make sure that everybody that has a life-threatening illness considered incurable can access holistic multidisciplinary care as they need.

I consider that compassion goes across all health care, not just palliative care, but I think the distinction is that people go to palliative care with the intent to try to prevent or alleviate suffering. That may not necessarily be the primary rationale for a dermatologist, a nurse in ICU, or a social worker engaged in child protection. If people see the prevention of suffering as part of compassionate care, then it follows that palliative care, by its nature, is compassionate care exemplified and demonstrated in the care we give to all—the prisoner, the IV drug user—irrespective of that person's background or whatever life situation they find themselves in.

Commentary

The common archetype of Christian compassion is that of the Good Samaritan. Another Christian story which reflects something of this chapter shared by Peter Hudson is that of St Francis of Assisi and the leper. It is told that early in his personal spiritual journey, Francis came across a leper with fulminating sores. Francis had a particular aversion to lepers, not least because of the disfigurement of this contagious disease and the ostracization from society which followed its diagnosis (Delio 2005. However, moved by the man' suffering, he dismounted his horse, gave the leper money, kissed his hand and moved on. Legend says that when he looked back, the leper had disappeared. The first biographer of Francis in the eleventh century, Thomas of Celano (see translated edition from 2000), noted that 'the holy lover of complete humility went to the lepers and lived with them, serving them most diligently for God's sake; and washing all foulness from them, he wiped away also the corruption of the ulcers (p.17).'

This not only evokes the medieval idea of hospice care for the poor and destitute, it also feeds into the more contemporary vision of care for dying people which aims to alleviate pain and suffering through dedicated supportive care. Inasmuch as compassion reflects our 'moved' response to the suffering other, it also suggests that the reason we reach out is that we are touched by the vulnerability of the other. Vulnerability is a complex issue and a term which, on the one hand, can express the reality of someone's situation or, on the other, be perceived as a value-laden label of criticism towards someone considered different or of less worth. Steinstra and Chochinov (2012) would argue that, although we could consider that everyone at end of life is vulnerable, its meaning in palliative care has come to represent distinct groups of marginalized people in society for whom access to services is obstructed. Amongst these are those with enduring mental illness, people with intellectual disability, the homeless, and those in prison. The challenges of providing palliative care to a prison population have been explored in the literature (Fletcher et al. 2014; Penrod et al. 2009). It has been argued that care for this group warrants a self-exploration of our own perspectives and views of the meaning and purpose of incarceration; in effect, is the purpose of incarceration exclusion or rehabilitation? Further, if working from a place of compassion in providing care, is that in any way mediated by the nature of the crime? Would a compassionate response be nuanced in some way if the prisoner was incarcerated for theft versus domestic violence or, as in this case, paedophilia? What is known is that the greater the degree of marginalization, the greater the limitation of access to palliative and end-of-life care (Chochinov & Steinstra 2012).

Vulnerability does not apply only to the recipient of care; there is evidence of how vulnerability can impact on those who give care. A Swedish study of qualified nurses' experience of working in a sitting service for dying patients showed that although they could see the benefit of the work they did, they also felt vulnerable in terms of decision-making and the impact these decisions had on people's experience of end of life (Wallerstedt et al. 2011). Conversely, a study by Malterud et al. (2009) found that doctors who expressed some level of personal vulnerability to the patient in relation to their interpretation and practice could gain a deeper understanding of the patient need and, in some cases, draw strength from that interaction. Gustin and Wagner (2013) conclude that compassion in care is neither demonstrated by just caregiving or by being present to another's suffering. It is 'a way of becoming and belonging together with another person where both are mutually engaged and where the caregiver compassionately is able to acknowledge both self and Other's vulnerability and dignity' (p. 175).

Compassionate caregiving is difficult. At difficult times, we seek refuge. If you have a faith practice, some aspect of that may supply the refuge you need at times of crisis. For others, it may be found through the aesthetics of life such as art, music, or nature. Within the Buddhist tradition, adherents may meditate on what is termed the three refuges: Buddha, Dharma, and Sangha. This encourages the person to reflect on the qualities of the Buddha—the need to show understanding to all beings, and, where possible, to do so within community.

The idea of the Sangha or community is an interesting one since it is the community which sustains, guides, and supports us in times of difficulty, and ensures that we adhere to the path. The idea of palliative care as a community is not unusual; it is part of the everyday vernacular. The community—be it the team, the profession, or the discipline—has the capacity to provide the refuge when facing our own or others' vulnerability in the face of life-threatening illness. It may be the anchor which enables us to reach out in often complex and harrowing situations, and to do that with the equanimity that those most vulnerable often need.

Reflections for practice

◆ From where do you access your support in the practice of palliative and end-of-life care?

◆ Is there a team which offers a Sangha for you to flourish in practice? If not, why may that be?

◆ How would you react to the case presented here? Are there other cases that would pose greater challenges for you in terms of practice? Why is that so?

Further reading

Chochinov HM, Steinstra D (2012) Vulnerability and palliative care. Palliative and Supportive Care, **10**, 1–2.

Delio I (2005) Compassion: living in the spirit of St Francis. Cincinnati, OH: Franciscan Media.

Fletcher A, Payne S, Waterman D, Turner M (2014) Palliative and end-of-life care in prisons in England and Wales—approaches taken to improve inequalities. BMJ Supportive Palliative Care, **4**, A19.

Gustin LW, Wagner L (2013) The butterfly effect of caring—clinical nursing teachers' understanding of self-compassion as a source to compassionate care. Scandinavian Journal of Caring Sciences, **27**(1), 175–183.

Malterud K, Friedriksen L, Gjerde MH (2009) When doctors experience their vulnerability as beneficial for the patients. Scandinavian Journal of Primary Health Care, **27**, 85–90.

Hanh TN (1995) Living Buddha, living Christ. New York: Riverhead.

Penrod J, Loed SJ, Smith CA (2009) Administrators' perspectives on changing practice in end-of-life care in a state prison system. Public Health Nursing, **31**(2), 99–108.

Stienstra D, Chochinov HM (2007) Palliative care for vulnerable populations. Palliative and Supportive Care, **10**, 37–42.

Thomas of Celano (2000) The first life of St Francis of Assisi. New York: Triangle.

Wallerstedt B, Benzein E, Andershead B (2011) Sharing living and dying: a balancing act between vulnerability and a sense of security: enrolled nurses' experience of working in the sitting service for dying patients at home. Palliative and Supportive Care, **9**, 295–303.

Chapter 16

Mari Lloyd-Williams— Community

Professor Mari Lloyd-Williams graduated from Leicester University medical school and completed her higher training in palliative medicine at University of Leicester Hospitals and LOROS Hospice. She was appointed consultant and honorary senior lecturer to the University of Leicester Hospitals Trust and LOROS Hospice in 2000. In 2002 she was appointed as senior lecturer at the University of Liverpool and in 2003 was promoted to a personal chair within the School of Population, Community and Behaviour in recognition of her research experience and portfolio. She has published over 100 papers and the seminal text *Psychosocial Issues in Palliative Care*, now in its second edition. She was also UK editor of the textbook *Palliative Medicine* by Walsh and colleagues, published initially in 2008.

She is lead and chair of the Academic Palliative and Supportive Care Studies Group within the University of Liverpool, which over the last five years has secured in excess of £5.3 million of research grant income, including the prestigious Supportive and Palliative Care research collaborative, as well as DoH and research council funding. The current research programme and portfolio include screening and interventions for depression; the development of randomized controlled trials in palliative care; and symptom burden in non-malignant disease, specifically for patients with dementia.

In 2007 she was appointed by the National Assembly for Wales onto the Higher Education Funding Council for Wales, and in 2008 she was appointed onto the UKHEAC committee chaired by Professor Sir John Tooke. A former member of fitness to practice panels for the General Medical Council, she is also chair and member of several external committees relating to health and education. She also lectures both nationally and internationally.

Foundations in palliative and end-of-life care

I was born in North Wales to a very loving, caring family. I am one of two children; I have a younger sister. I was brought up on a farm in a very rural community, where the local chapel was part of my being. I was brought up in a three-generation family. When I was three my maternal grandfather died and my grandmother came to live with us. I was not unique in having grandparent living with us. When I look back, I think that was a hugely formative part of my upbringing. My parents were very involved in the community; it was not just about being involved on a Sunday. As a small child, I was aware that lots of people came to see my parents for different sorts of help and advice. I suppose that compassion was there from a very early age. My mother was very busy helping my father and not always at home, so my sister and I cared for our grandmother. At the time I was not aware of it but that probably shaped me and had a huge influence on my life.

I went to medical school in Leicester, which was a hugely happy experience and very different for me from a small parish in North Wales. I don't come from a medical background at all. From a very young age I can remember wanting to do operations on my dolls, much to my sister's horror. I am sure the fact that I was quite exposed to hospitals as a child was significant, certainly with my grandmother and because of my mother's involvement with the local community. I would be taken to visit various people in hospital because there was nobody else to look after my sister and me. Being in Leicester where half of the community were from a South Asian background was amazing because North Wales was traditionally a very white area and I absolutely loved Leicester—celebrating the fact that we are all very similar when we think we are dissimilar.

I was in Leicester for quite some time. I did my specialist palliative care training there and obtained a consultant post. I then moved to Liverpool, initially for a senior lecturer post, and was then promoted to a chair. I have been in Liverpool now for ten years. As well as my academic role, I work clinically. I have outpatient clinics at the hospice. I do some work with the hepatobiliary team as well as hospital support. I think the clinical work is essential, that is what I trained for. The academic work is important but research has to be clinically embedded and of clinical value to be worth doing at all.

The compassionate practitioner

I hope that I am a compassionate practitioner. I think it is essential, because for so many patients we meet, their care has been clinically sound but not compassionate. Many of our patients at referral tell us stories of non-compassionate care. Compassion is essential for all doctors, not just in hospice and palliative care. It is really something we need to embed in training for all health care professionals because it does not matter how trivial a patient's admission seems to us, we do not know what that illness means to them in the context of what else is going on in their lives. If you have personally received health care, you know that the compassionate approach just makes such a difference. It certainly does with family members. It does mean putting yourself in another's shoes, thinking 'How would this feel for that person and their family?' Patients bring their physical problems to clinic but you cannot help any physical problems if you do not address the social, psychological, and spiritual as well. Having that level of engagement is crucial. I feel incredibly privileged that I have worked with teams of people who were deeply compassionate. There is something hugely supportive and affirmative working with people who share the same ethos. If there are difficult situations you have got that mutual support and understanding.

I would say most health care professionals do have a compassionate approach, especially in palliative care; it translates to your daily life as well. I don't mean to suggest that a palliative care practitioner has deeper compassion than other colleagues. I worked in psychiatry for a year. I think psychiatrists get a bit of a bad press. I worked with some hugely compassionate psychiatrists who were just wonderful and gave the patients such compassionate care. It was almost humbling to be present. We have this archetypal image of surgeons, and yet I can think of some surgeons that I have worked with who stand out within their clinical team for their compassion. That must be quite difficult because they often don't have that nurturing support from their colleagues. Perhaps those who go into hospice and palliative care have a greater sense of that compassionate nurturing.

I think compassion is integral to the way we communicate with each other. You can tell so much about how person even in the way they say hello. It does worry me that we spend thousands of pounds each year trying to teach our medical students communication skills and we don't seem to get it right.

I always remember being with a medical student visiting a very young patient with a poor prognosis. I said, 'If you had been in my chair, what would you have said to the patient?' She said very matter-of-factly, 'I can feel your pain.' The way it was said it was like 'I am catching a bus.' It just meant nothing. When I asked why she said that, she replied, 'That is what we were taught.' I do worry that we select our medical students very much on academic criteria, but perhaps we do not give enough attention to compassion, especially in our society where people seem so disengaged from community support.

I think our life experiences influence our ability to be compassionate, depending on the circumstance. I think it is something innate shaped by life experiences. I worked with a lovely nurse colleague who did have a feeling that sometimes nurses became less compassionate at the end of their careers because they had almost given too much compassion earlier. Yet I worked with some amazing nurses who at the age of 65 were as compassionate, possibly more so, on their last day of work as on their first. I think it is that nurturing of compassion through working with others who share the same way of thinking. I think if you are working more in isolation that must be much more difficult.

Increasingly, I think we see hospice and palliative care providing that support to people at the end of their lives. So many people who don't have family or a faith-based community don't have any links. People in our generation will be looking for those links more because I think the professional middle classes struggle with compassion themselves. Certainly they want it when it comes to their personal experiences.

A case exemplar

I think of one particular case of a man who, from the age of 18 to about 60, had been in a psychiatric hospital. I think at the age of 18 he had some sort of breakdown, had been admitted to a psychiatric hospital, and had to stay there as people did in those days. During that time his parents had died. He was the youngest of a large family, but had little support from them. The NHS focus on community mental health meant that the hospital closed, and he was told, You are free to go home.

Of course he had no home and ended up in a flat with limited social support. He really struggled. He was in that flat two to three years, living with severe mental health problems, and then he developed colorectal cancer. He was admitted to hospital, had surgery and an oncology intervention, and then was referred to hospice day care. The oncologist saw that although this man probably did not have a terminal diagnosis at that time, he needed more in the way of support. I think that came from a place of compassion.

I started seeing him in my clinic. In those days, people could come to day care several days a week for quite a long time. I think hospice day care offers so much to people who are on the margins of our society, who probably do not experience any level of care, compassion, and love anywhere else. He really was a very needy person. He did not have any social skills, no friends. He ate out in cafes. The nurse in charge of the day care looked out for him. She went around to charity shops looking for clothes for him because his self-care was really poor. Day care only closed Christmas Day, Boxing Day, and New Year's Day, and she made sure that he was in on Christmas Eve and the days between Christmas and New Year's as she knew how isolated he was.

He used to send me these little snippets, three or four days a week, always first-class post, just to tell me 'I have been shopping to . . .' or 'I had a cup of coffee in . . .' —whatever. You might call them a paper Twitter. He would send about 20 Christmas cards, one a week from August. I think he desperately wanted us to know he was still there. He was scared of us forgetting about him.

I remember him telling me that having cancer was the best thing that ever happened to him. He would come to my clinic and always arrive about eight o'clock on the bus. I would see him and there was a little snack bar and someone would make sure he had some tea or coffee and he would have a bit of lunch and he would speak to everybody. About four o'clock, after he had his tea and cake, he would go home. I think that day probably gave him that element of sustenance support and care that probably allowed him to live.

He would find any excuse to come to the hospice. I actually ended up seeing him for about three to four years. I had various people asking me why this person was coming to my clinic on a monthly basis. He did not fit the stereotype of our traditional terminal hospice patient, and if it had been now he probably would not have got through the door. When I think of him, he epitomizes what I suppose is a very traditional model of compassionate hospice care. There were no strings attached, no questions asked—we will love and care for you. He was on the periphery of every community. I spent a lot of time phoning various social service departments to try to access more support for him—but he did not fit. The mental health team were only able to intervene if he was a danger to himself or others, which he wasn't. He could not access the elderly mental health team because he had a chronic mental illness and not dementia. The GP service changed and he saw different people in the surgery, usually the locum or the trainee. The hospice really was his only source of continuity.

Then, one day, he did not turn up for an appointment. He would usually write before his clinic appointment, 'I am coming to see you on Monday', or 'two days before I am coming to see you.' It was quite obvious that something had happened. We found out after a week or two that he had been admitted acutely into hospital with pneumonia and had died. We felt very sad that he had not been able to die in the hospice that meant so much to him, because his disease was not classified as terminal. That said, we had a great sense that we really had made a big difference to somebody who did not fit anywhere else. He had been very fortunate to have had that compassionate oncologist. The oncology teams are so busy, it is probable that no one would have identified this poor man as in need of a bit of extra support. He was fortunate that he had an oncologist who referred him to the hospice. He was fortunate the model of hospice day care at that time gave him the possibility of support. Despite a lot of opposition from both medical and nursing staff, we fought to keep him in the clinical system. That to me demonstrates true compassionate care.

It worries me slightly the way hospice care is changing. If he had been referred to a hospice today, I am not sure he would have been accepted, because his main issue was his mental illness, not his cancer. We can all be criticized for providing this Rolls-Royce care for the few, but sometimes those few are the very ones that need it because they never get it anywhere else. You can be open to a lot of criticism from colleagues, particularly where the specialist palliative care service may consider that they do not deal with things like mental illness. Of course, you cannot care for everyone, but sometimes you should not be afraid to reach out. Every service has to evolve, and clearly there are serious issues about the fact that you can only provide a limited service for a very small number of people. I think we just need to be careful. I strongly believe in day care. I think hospice day care is very much thought of as the Cinderella of the hospice, somewhere you go for a cup of tea for all the good it does. I think we negate the compassionate care it offers and the difference it makes. We need to hold on to this. We may think that because we are providing an acute service we cannot be compassionate, and that is simply not so.

We did some research here with the Intensive Therapy Unit (ITU). More patients die in ITU than die in hospice. Yet, by and large, carers did not describe compassionate care. There were many issues about the fact that they felt hurried when life support was being switched off. Someone actually died while we were there. They were waiting for a son to come and the nurse said, 'Look, this has gone on long enough; when is he coming? We need the bed.' Of course, there were also good examples but, especially around issues of organ donation, retrieving the organ seemed far more important than the care of the patient or the care of the family at the time. So I wonder what makes care in a hospice different to care in ITU? Both are usually small units, with a high ratio of staff and a multidisciplinary team working, and death is a frequent occurrence. True compassion is not disease- or symptom-specific. It should be across-the-board.

Fostering sustainable compassion

I think recruitment is key. I think that is so important: whom we recruit and how we recruit them. The questions about 'What draws you here? What will sustain you?' are really important. Clearly we don't want all the people to be the same. You need to have a mix of people for it to work. I think role modelling is extremely important. In the day care setting I discussed earlier, the person in charge was quite formidable but was deeply, deeply compassionate, a lovely person. The matron was, again, quite formidable, but would do anything for the patients or her staff and volunteers. There was a tremendous sense that you were all part of a big jigsaw. You fitted into that jigsaw and that jigsaw was important to the patient.

I think strong, compassionate leadership is definitely what is needed, and that people need to see that it is alright to be compassionate. It is not weak and woolly. It is something that is of vital importance to our patients—of the same importance as making sure you get the opioid doses right. It really does make a huge difference to them. It does not mean you necessarily need extra resources or time. In fact, if you can deliver compassionate care well, you almost can be quicker, because people are more satisfied. It is when people are dissatisfied that they perhaps demand more of your time, because they are not getting what they want or need.

Cicely Saunders said, 'The way that care is given can reach the most hidden places and give space for unexpected development.' I think that is a very profound statement, and it is so true. Delivering compassionate care actually sustains you because you have the feeling that you have done your very best. People I know who have really struggled felt that they had failed in some way because of their organizational structures. I think that is where the team approach is vital: the fact that you are working with other people focused towards the same cause. That allows you to receive support which is so important.

I think palliative care has been very much within the walls of the hospice. Palliative care teams in hospitals have not really developed to the same extent. I think there is a lot of work to be done there, really.

For sustainability, the hospice and palliative care approach needs to be available to all people, and not just at the very end of life. I am particularly concerned that the way we treat and care for our older people is often less than compassionate. We need to consider how we care for our elders, and if we brought compassion to bear in that question. I think it would transform our health care system. It would really make a difference.

Commentary

Community would seem to be a common thread running through palliative and end-of-life care, and its importance frames much of the experience shared here by Professor Mari Lloyd-Williams. We speak about the palliative care community, which gives a sense of a body of people with similar aspirations and goals. At one point in her selected letters relating to the early formulation of ideas about hospice and palliative care, In her selected writings (Clark 2005), Cicely Saunders mused on the idea of hospice care being delivered by a community of people living and working together in a lay religious context where prayer held an important space in the care of the patient and the community itself. Clearly, this links back to the earliest iterations of hospice care delivered through the care of religious communities, not only in the Christian tradition. Maria Rosa Mendocal's (2002) critique of how cultural tolerance between Jews, Muslims, and Christians in early medieval Spain engendered new and creative ways of coexistence also reflected the way that those most vulnerable in society were treated and respected. Contemporary interfaith dialogues equally voice the need to have a shared understanding of how to reach out to those most vulnerable, because we are ostensibly indivisible (http://www.charterforcompassion.org)—as Mari Lloyd-Williams puts it, 'Celebrating the fact that we are all very similar when we think we are dissimilar.'

The case presented by Mari Lloyd-Williams considers the issue of people with enduring mental illness, frequently marginalized within society and health care overall, and one of the groups least likely to access palliative services. In *The Evolution of God*, Robert Wright (2010) argues that compassion is contingent on the belief that we are willing to comprehend the world from the viewpoint of the other person, and without the ability to do that, compassion fails. All the rhetoric that is linked to the language and formation of compassionate practice (*being with, reaching out*, etc.) stems from the fundamental principle that we are genuinely interested in what happens to the other person and want to try to see what it like to be them. In the case exemplar, we see many 'communities' (mental health, older person care, community care) who, with every good intention, have become silos where those in greatest need do not fit by virtue of their difference or failure to meet specific criteria. Such is the case here.

The French anthropologist Marc Augé (1995) has commented that hospitals and health care settings are rapidly becoming '*non-lieu*' (non-places). By this he means that there is no space created which allows the sick person to feel that they are 'dwelling' rather than simply 'passing through'. Our modern world favours a rapid response rather than a measured nurturing over time. The latter may be more meaningful in the delivery of palliative care, but that requires a reflective stance on who we were and what we have become. We, as a practice community, need to take time to reflect on the messages that the early hospice movement gave us and consider how they still apply today. The idea of a compassionate community is not new to palliative care. The work of Professor Allan Kellehear (2013) and his passionate belief that care for people at end of life should arise from a community-orientated public health model is well referenced. It is perhaps timely to make sense of what compassion means for us both as practitioners and a community of practice.

Reflections for practice

- ◆ What lessons from the early view of hospice care are still relevant to contemporary practice today? What can sustain them? What challenges them?

- ◆ To what extent do you perceive palliative care as a community? Is that a helpful descriptor in the way you see palliative care practised?

- ◆ How well has palliative and end-of-life care embraced a palliative-care-for-all approach that extends to those who may consider themselves marginalized from society? What have we got right? What have we yet to learn?

Further reading

Augé M (1995) Non-places: introduction to an anthropology of supermodernity (transl. J Howe). London: Verso.

Clark D (2005) Cicely Saunders: selected writings, 1958–2004. Oxford: Oxford University Press.

Kearney M (2007) Mortally wounded: stories of soul pain, death, and healing (2nd ed.). New Orleans, LA: Spring Journal.

Kellehear A (2013) Compassionate communities: end-of-life care as everyone's responsibility. QJM: An International Journal of Medicine, **106**, 1071–1075.

Koffman J, Camps M (2008) 'No way in': including disadvantaged population and patient groups at end-of-life. In S Payne et al. (eds) Palliative care nursing: principles and evidence for practice (2nd ed.). 362–382.

Lloyd-Williams M (2009) Psychosocial care in palliative care (2nd ed.). Oxford: Oxford University Press.

Mendocal MR (2002) The ornament of the world: how Muslims, Jews and Christians created a culture of tolerance in Medieval Spain. Boston: Little Brown.

Wright R (2010) The evolution of God. Boston: Back Bay Books.

Walsh, D, Foley KM, Caraceni A, Fainsinger R, Glare P, Goh C, Lloyd-Williams M, Nunez-Olarte J, Radbruch L (2008) Palliative Medicine, Expert Consult. Philadelphia, WB Saunders Company.

Chapter 17

Anne Merriman—
Interconnectedness

Dr Anne Merriman was born into an Irish Catholic family in Liverpool, where she spent her childhood. She went to Ireland in 1953 where she joined a religious order, the Medical Missionaries of Mary, and was enrolled in medical school at University College Dublin. After qualification in 1963, she completed an internship in the International Missionary Training Hospital in Drogheda. She subsequently worked in Ireland, Nigeria, and Scotland, completing her MRCPI and MRCP (UK Edinburgh) as well as diplomas in child health and tropical medicine. Later she was made fellow of the Royal College of Physicians in both Ireland and Edinburgh. After specializing in geriatric medicine, she identified and encouraged meeting the needs for palliative care among the elderly in her practice in Whiston Hospital in Merseyside. She subsequently worked in Malaysia and then Singapore, where she developed the idea of affordable powdered morphine reconstituted into liquid for use in the home, which she later took to Africa.

Anne Merriman has spent 33 years working in Africa. In 1992, she founded Hospice Africa with a vision to bring palliative care to all in need in Sub Saharan Africa. The model was commenced in Uganda (Hospice Africa Uganda HAU)) in 1993. The model introduced a palliative and end-of-life care programme, based on control of severe pain through access to affordable morphine, which is now freely available in Uganda. This has since been introduced to many other countries in Africa. Currently, as Director of International Programmes, she has supported similar initiatives, adapted to each country's economic and cultural needs, across the continent of Africa, including Tanzania, Nigeria, Cameroon, Malawi, Sierra Leone, Ethiopia, Zambia, Rwanda, and Sudan, and, more recently, initiatives in Togo and DRC.

She is the author of *Audacity to Love: The Story of Hospice Africa: Bringing Hope and Peace for the Dying*. In addition to many other honours bestowed on her, she received the MBE in 2003 for palliative care services to Uganda and was a 2014 nominee for the Nobel Peace Prize.

Foundations in palliative and end-of-life care

I trained as a doctor in UCD, Ireland, and completed my final training there and later in Edinburgh as fellow of the Royal College of Physicians. The first time I was aware that there was a need for some special care for people at end of life was when I was in geriatric medicine in the UK. After ten years in Nigeria, I spent eight years working in Merseyside and Manchester, before going back out to developing countries again. I found that there were a lot of people in long-term care being kept alive and suffering a lot. There was no adequate pain control in the 70s. Palliative care had not been introduced into the Mersey region. I started reading the books by Dame Cicely Saunders and Robert Twycross, and used their methods for pain control, teaching it to the geriatric teams and eventually, on request, to the surgical and medical teams. We then invited Dame Cicely to come to Whiston Hospital, which she eventually did in 1981. This was hugely popular. They came from all over the region. When she saw the need, she gave the first two Macmillan nurses to St Helen's and Knowsley District.

I went from there to Malaysia and then to Singapore. The services were all based on home care in those early days, trying to keep people where they wanted to die, mainly in their own homes. We needed pain control in the home, so with the pharmacists, we made up a formula—morphine powder, water, a dye, and a preservative—just these four ingredients. It was very cheap—cost only $1 for ten days' treatment and kept the patient completely pain-free. Before that, only 'Brompton's cocktail' was available, which contained many additives. We wanted just pure oral morphine that we could give to patients in their own homes.

When I was in Singapore, the wife of a BBC correspondent, Ruth Wooldridge, a nurse herself, set up a trust to start a hospice in Nairobi, Kenya. She had seen people coming home from hospitals and dying in the community in agony and realized there had to be an answer to this. One of the trust board members was with Robert Twycross on a visit to Singapore. They were looking for their first medical director, saw what I was doing, and invited me to go there for interview. When I arrived in Nairobi, I couldn't believe what I was seeing. The strongest analgesic for people at home was codeine. Very few were accessing curative treatment. We were seeing terrible suffering with little relief from the step 1 and occasionally step 2 analgesics. Those in severe pain who could not afford the simplest of analgesics were left to suffer terrible pain. I was offered the post but said I would only go if they brought in powdered morphine for reconstitution. Within six months they were using it and I joined them.

Nairobi made me realize two things. Firstly, hospitals were sending people home saying, 'There is nothing more we can do for you.' Even I had done this in

Nigeria. But we had never looked into the homes to see what was happening! Secondly, I realized that this was the case not just in Nairobi, but also all over Africa. In 1992, the only palliative care available was in Zimbabwe and South Africa, which had well-structured palliative care, largely for the white community. They were moving to incorporate it within the black African communities. Zimbabwe already had a large number of African HIV/AIDS patients on their programme. Nairobi was different. It was the first one started for all in need (mainly the black Africans) by a white person.

Following a request from several countries to bring them a service similar to Nairobi's, I realized that the other countries were ready for palliative care, and I was inspired to try to meet these needs. I had written an article about the work in Nairobi, describing one case only, for the journal *Contact* from the Christian Medical Commission in Geneva, which went out free to African countries. This edition was dedicated to palliative care and edited by Dame Cicely Saunders. I then realized a vision to embrace all those in need in Africa, and recognized that this might be done from a model which could be adapted to the cultures and economies in different countries.

I knew such a model would need to be able to train people so that it would reach the whole of Africa. I went to the UK for a year to try to get a group together to support this vision financially. In 1993, we did a feasibility study to see where we would place this organization. Nairobi did not want to take more on board, as they had enough to do with so many sick in their densely populated city.

We had heard from about seven countries asking for us to help them develop a similar service, and we tried to reach out to them, but in those days it was fairly hard to get in touch, as it was all through posted correspondence—e-mail was not yet established. Moi University in Eldoret, Kenya, wanted us to start there, but Nairobi Hospice were concerned that funding would be a problem if we set up in another part of Kenya. So in early 1993, after visiting four countries in the feasibility study, we chose Uganda. They were just out of the war and had the confidence of the international community, so we hoped we might raise the money. Singapore knew what I was capable of doing and gave me enough money for three team members for three months. We began in September: a nurse who had worked with me in Nairobi, Fazal Mbaraka, and I. She was of Asian descent, born and brought up in Kenya, and spoke the languages. Sadly, her father was murdered during the time I was raising money. I had left her in Uganda to set up things. She was only with me for about three months of the service starting and had to return to support her grieving family. So then I started looking for local dedicated nurses. The first nurse, Rose, is now the country director of the Palliative Care Association of Uganda, which follows up those we train and ensures morphine distribution in Uganda. The second nurse, Martha, is still with HAU after 20 years.

We started care and training at the same time—that was terribly important. We started teaching undergraduate doctors immediately, so, since 1994, all newly qualified doctors are trained in and understand palliative medicine.

When I look back it was easy compared to today. The donors trusted that we knew what we were doing in those days. Now there is so much that the donors demand—you can spend more time at meetings than seeing patients. Then, we saw what was necessary and just went ahead and did it. Today, we have 112 Ugandan team members, looking after 1,700 patients across three sites, mainly in their own homes. Our main donor, USAID, is cutting back; next year their funding ends, so we are having some difficulty. Out of a population of 35 million, we estimate about 200,000 require palliative care in Uganda at the moment. Fifty per cent have cancer and about 50 per cent have HIV/AIDS: 30 per cent of our patients are HIV-positive only and 20 per cent have cancer and are HIV-positive. We ask if they wish to be tested; some don't, because when you are dying of cancer you don't want to have a double upset by knowing you are HIV-positive as well. So we can only try to estimate it clinically within the WHO guidelines.

The compassionate practitioner

One of the biggest problems today is that compassion is gone from general medicine. I feel that palliative care has something to offer the whole of medicine, not just the patients in palliative care. Compassion comes from being able to recognize the needs of the patient: that means listening and adapting to the changing needs of a patient as you are looking after them. Not only listening, but if you don't know the answers, being able to admit you don't know, seek further advice and, if necessary, try to help them in other ways. We may have to relate to other organizations and teams to help us in these different areas.

For me, our compassion comes through in our ethos. The ethos is based on three main pillars. First, the patient and family is the centre of all we do, whether we sweep the floor or whether we are medically seeing the patients. Second, we care for each other so that if we have problems, either inside or outside of hospice, we can talk to somebody and receive a compassionate response from that person so that we don't go out all upset and angry and project that onto the patient. Third, we accept that we cannot do everything as one organization and we need the help of others. If only we could recognize that we are not in competition with each other for funding or anything else! We all contribute. In Uganda, as different agencies we founded became independent, they began to see us as a rival. I feel that this ethos of collaboration is terribly important for us in palliative care if it is going to move forward in Africa. When we ask people, many of whom do not have access to morphine or other medications, what they have learnt from our training, they say, 'I learnt that I could listen to the patient—that I could actually sit down on the bed and talk to them eye to eye.' That is so important to the care of patients.

They could not do that before. We go back to being human beings. When they were at home in the villages they cared for each other. Now, we take people and we train them in medicine and nursing but we risk dehumanizing them, hiding behind our uniform and our superiority. I just think that medicine in particular is such a proud and arrogant profession. To think we are above anybody else is really sad. We can't really help them unless we can get with them at the same level and realize our shared humanity. If we are the only profession with a success rate measure in cure then we are the only ones with 100 per cent failure rate because everyone is going to die.

Making money is the other big thing. We see patients who have been to many, many doctors, just like in the Gospel—the woman who had been to many doctors. They have never told the truth; they always say they will do more because they would get more money. Some people have not even been examined. The first time they are examined may be when they get to us and we find they have something very obvious, like a huge liver, because they have never even had a hand put on the area. It is really sad. There is a lot of bribery and corruption at all levels in Africa, and Uganda is now one of the highest. The big donors are more into numbers. For example, USAID focuses completely on HIV and they want you to have a large number of HIV patients. We have more than 2,000 organizations in Uganda with the name HIV or AIDS in their name. USAID often give large salaries. They like to pay people to come on courses. If you come on a course for the money you are not going to be a good palliative care person. We have to look very carefully at the reasons and agendas. Training has also changed considerably. Hands-on practical training is less and there is much more on measurement, audits, etc. In 1993 when we started, nobody asked us had we done an audit on this, that, and the other. You explained a case, you told them, and that was it. But it has really changed.

People's lives change when they come on home visits. Every case needs compassion and anybody on a home visit will see a team exhibiting compassion for the patient. Sometimes it is difficult to get that quiet time with the patient when they can confide in you, and that is something we stress—team members need to create that time with the patient. The caring approach is at the essence of it, that is part of compassion. The caring person has to be empathetic, able to understand and adapt to the changing condition over time because some of the patients often die very quickly. Others don't die at all. We care for a 17-year-old girl with paraplegia and we have been trying to support her in different ways for 11 years. She has recently passed nine O levels, in spite of being carried to school by her classmates and living at home with no electricity.

What is really amazing is that no matter whether they have killed a grandmother or robbed a bank, when it comes to dying the patients know there is a compassionate God and they very much want that spiritual link. I have yet to meet a patient in Uganda who does not believe in God. Everyone believes in a God that is going to forgive him or her. That is a compassionate God. Unfortunately, the Catholic Church here is traditional and very 'pre-Vatican'. There is a sign at a local school, where one of the little girls from my house goes, saying 'First: all children must fear God'—I asked them to take it down. Why are they teaching the kids to fear God? They should know a loving God, not fear him.

A case exemplar

I have two short but similar cases from the very early days. The first woman was in the ward in Nsambya Hospital. We were working from our house, seeing patients in the front room and going into the hospital and patients' homes. This woman, Mary, was in the gynaecology ward, in a kind of outhouse. All the other patients had disappeared because she smelt so bad. She was the only one in the ward! She had developed cancer of the rectum and had surgery in May and a colostomy fitted. When it came time for her to go home, she could not pay her bill and so they kept her in. Her husband had disappeared. She had five children. She had to go back to her mother.

While at home she developed a growth in her lymph glands in the groin. A traditional healer opened them, thought it was an abscess, and she was stinking from that. Mary had been readmitted again in September. We were able to manage the smell. The nurses did not know about metronidazole or how to control smell. She was very thin and debilitated. We controlled her pain; we controlled the smell and got her home. We followed her up at home. Her big problem was that her mother had five other adult children who had all died of AIDS. So the grandmother was looking after nine young children. She was breaking stones to make money. We got a group of volunteers from Holland to pay for the stones for the grandmother to break up so she could manage the kids and school fees. One of Mary's children had HIV and died very young. Our patient died within six weeks.

At the same time we had a second woman, Margaret, who had had a colostomy three years previously, for the same reason, cancer of the rectum. Her partner and father of her children was a doctor who moved to South Africa.

After her colostomy he did not want anything to do with her. She was on her own. She lived for about six months after we met her. The difference was that Mary had HIV and she should never have been operated on because she could not heal. Before she died, the rectum and colostomy opened and fell into the abdominal cavity. Her body was falling to pieces because her resistance was so low. I think that the most compassionate response goes beyond the patient, because we were able to advise the surgeons to do a HIV test before they operated on a patient, and if the CD count was very low, reconsider because of the consequences of such complex situations afterwards. In those days it was terrible—people were dying all over the place. Of course, this was before ARVs (anti-retrovirals) came in 2003. One in seven had 'slim disease' and would be dead within a year.

We saw some terrible situations: we saw young pregnant women with Kaposi's sarcoma, which had never occurred in women before AIDS. Some would get cryptococcal meningitis and die, and the baby would die because there was no breast milk. It was so sad. Only the few lucky ones got to us. The rest died in their communities. Having community volunteers to identify people in pain is so important. Fifty-seven per cent of people never see health workers in Uganda. In Ethiopia it was 85 per cent. We talk as if everybody is going to get to the hospital, but they don't. Somebody has to recognize that and help them in their communities.

Fostering sustainable compassion

I think our team members are good at sustaining themselves but we have certain things within our teams to try to maintain the spirit. Keeping people together is important. We are divided into the academic institute, the clinical side, and then administration. We hold a monthly meeting where we hear from each group what they're doing. We have an annual day of reflection, to see where we are with our own God and our relationship with hospice and our patients. We also have a round table where we socialize over drinks and if you speak about hospice you have to put money in a box for the next round! Every morning we begin with a short prayer and then discuss the day ahead. I go back to the ethos. We now call it the ethos for hospices in Africa and try to apply it to the new hospital-based home care teams. Hospitals are bureaucratic and struggle to absorb that ethos. So it is very hard to get the ethos into hospital home care teams. If you haven't got the ethos you are not going to get that spirit of compassion— the ethos is the way back to hospitality towards our patients.

I would like to see the whole spirit of palliative care getting through to all health care professionals. I think we shouldn't isolate palliative care. It is cross-cutting.

People don't only die of cancer and HIV/AIDS. They die of renal failure, heart failure, and all the rest. If only we could only get that spirit of compassion into the medical profession from the start. One way would be to get a medical student to adopt a family in their first year and watch that family go through, seeing the life and death in the family. Following them up in different ways each year, then they can really understand what it is like. In Africa, every country and culture is different. I am not sure that being taught out of Western textbooks helps, but that is what they will be examined on. At least, in Uganda, we are getting them examined in palliative care as well.

I have just come from Paris where we have been reviewing last year's Francophone courses. They couldn't believe in Africa such a model could exist—where everybody works so closely together and even though we didn't speak the same language, there was such a closeness so they could see that medicine was not only just treating the patient, it was actually seeing the patients' problems, and that they could identify them and that they could care for them. For them it was eye-opening. You cannot give holistic care with people screaming with pain. Human rights activists suggest that to leave someone in pain is akin to torture. We have got to realize that. Yet none of the Francophone countries have affordable oral morphine.

I think for me it is easy to work in Uganda because people believe in God, in some way. The traditional religions believe in God as a Supreme Being as well as their ancestors. As health workers, the ability to recognize when they need help with their spirituality, either from us or from somebody else, is important. There is a lot of guilt associated with the religions in Africa as well, and that can be very painful to talk about. I find it difficult when sometimes people are condemned for talking about God but, of course, if people do not want to talk about God, then you don't. People are spiritual beings so you have to be willing to approach that as well.

I think my own compassion was developed as a child from seeing compassionate parents, but I think also that if you have read the gospels you see that Christ was compassionate. Christ in the New Testament is quite different to the approach in the Old Testament, which was not so compassionate at all. I think the definition you give from Henri Nouwen shows that he was a very compassionate person. I think compassion is catching. I think if you work with compassionate people it rubs off.

Commentary

Trystan Owain Hughes (2013) argues for 'radical compassion in practice' (p. 65). Radical compassion moves us beyond the awareness of another's suffering to an active engagement to alleviate that suffering in whatever way we can. The root of radical compassion is based in mutual respect and togetherness. Looking at the cases which Anne Merriman shares, there is a clear call for the need to work together; to focus less on what makes us different and more what makes us the same. The second case in particular demonstrates why the feeling of compassion towards someone who is suffering is not sufficient. The action—in this case, advising the surgeons of the best course of action in the case of a HIV/AIDS patient before clinical decisions regarding intervention are made—demonstrates the argument of Owain Hughes most clearly. Both Christian and Buddhist perspectives on compassion would see this interconnectedness between people and their world as an essential part of compassionate practice. Joan Halifax, the US based Buddhist scholar, refers to 'non-referential' compassion—a sense that we aspire to heal suffering because we are all connected in some way (Halifax 2011). Such compassion is not directed to any one individual. Rather, it is universal and reaches out beyond the encounter between self and other. Reaching out in the spirit of seeking connection would seem to encapsulate the vision of Anne Merriman's work across Africa. Palliative care has moved towards embracing this wider vision of care beyond cancer. The current focus of palliative care principles beyond diagnosis or disease reflects the mutuality of relationship between health care practitioners, irrespective of discipline. It is grounded in a profound belief in the desire to heal and alleviate suffering wherever possible. Moreover, it acknowledges that our interconnectedness as a professional team is the greatest gift we offer the patient and family to assist them to reach their goals for care.

Reflections for practice

- Consider in what ways the palliative care practitioner reaches out to connect in compassionate ways to alleviate suffering.
- To what extent are you able to demonstrate that in your professional life and clinical practice?
- What are the challenges to developing an interconnected approach to palliative and end-of-life care?

Further reading

Downing J, Leng M, Namukwaya E, Murray S, Atieno M, Grant L (2014) Lessons from four countries in sub-Saharan African in defining and developing integrated models of palliative care. BMJ Supportive and Palliative Care, 4(1), A82–83.

Famoroti TO, Fernandes L, Chima SC (2013) Stigmatization of people living with HIV/AIDS by healthcare workers at a tertiary hospital in KwaZulu-Natal, South Africa: a cross-sectional descriptive study. BMC Medical Ethics, 14, Suppl 1, S6.

Halifax J (2011) The precious necessity of compassion. Journal of Pain and Symptom Management, **41**(1), 146–152.

Kuah-Pearce KE (2014) Understanding suffering and giving compassion: the reach of socially engaged Buddhism in China. Anthropological Medicine, **21**(1), 27–42.

Owain Hughes T (2013) The compassion quest. London: SPCK.

Soyannwo O (2014) Pain management in sub-Saharan Africa: innovative approaches to improving access. Pain Management, **4**(1), 5–7.

Chapter 18

Daniela Mosoiu—
Compassionate love

Dr Daniela Mosoiu graduated from medical school in 1991 and worked in medical oncology and palliative care. In 1995, she became part of the Hospice Casa Sperantei team—the first hospice in Romania. In 1997, the Study Centre for Palliative Care was opened in Brasov and she became responsible for education and continued professional education for medical and allied health care professionals. She has contributed to the training of over 10,000 professionals within Romania and abroad, and became a national trainer in palliative care, accredited by health ministry. In this role, she has fostered greater palliative care education opportunities for Eastern Europe, supported by the Open Society Institute. In 2013, University Transilvania Brasov created the first palliative care academic position in Romania and Dr Mosoiu was appointed as associate professor, coordinating the palliative care multidisciplinary master's programme.

She is co-founder of the National Association of Palliative Care. In 2000, she headed the working group that brought recognition of palliative care as a medical sub-specialty in Romania, and at present she is national coordinator for palliative care sub-specialty for doctors. As vice president in the National Commission for Palliative Care and Pain Therapy, she contributed to changing the legal framework regarding prescription and use of opioids in Romania, and is in the process of implementing the new legislation.

In 2008, she created a partnership between the health ministry and Hospice Casa Sperantei in order to develop a national strategy. She holds a large teaching portfolio and has been an invited speaker to conferences and congresses throughout Romania and internationally. She has published several books on palliative care and, until 2013, was a board director of the Worldwide Palliative Care Alliance.

Foundations in palliative and end-of-life care

I started working in palliative care in 1995 after I finished my training as an oncologist. In Romania, even working as an oncologist, 75 per cent of the patients that you saw were patients with advanced cancer. So a lot of patients coming for their cancer treatment were patients with advanced disease with many complex symptoms. Some of them were dying in hospital while, at the same time, getting chemotherapy and not really receiving proper care. I found it quite distressing, but I didn't know at that time that there was another way to care. By chance, I started to work with the hospice, not knowing exactly what it meant. I agreed that I would work with them for three months as a trial period and I am still here, 19 years later.

I started doing home care. We were the first organization doing this kind of hospice care. By hospice, of course, I don't mean a building but rather a philosophy of care. In Romania, we make no distinction between palliative care and hospice care. We use these words interchangeably. We were quite a small team when I joined—just ten people including administration. It has now grown quite large and we offer care in the capital, Bucharest, and in the city of Brasov. We also have two mobile teams in the rural area of Brasov district. Hospice Casa Sperantei was set up as a British-Romanian foundation by Graham Perolls, a British man who had lost his father due to cancer and who first set up a hospice home care service in Dartford, Kent. He had strong links to Brasov, and in 1989 he visited the local oncology hospital where he saw a young man dying in pain. He wanted to know how best to help, and because he had experience of setting up a hospice in the UK, he agreed to do that in Brasov, and we opened in 1992. Now we are part of the Hospices of Hope network with branches in the UK, USA, Romania, Moldova, and Serbia.

Originally our head nurse was a woman from the UK who volunteered to work with us in Romania for two years. Today the team is fully Romanian. We have now 160 people employed and working across the service. We propose to open a new hospice in Bucharest in the autumn and develop two further rural community teams.

Graham was visionary. We both saw the need to develop an education programme, more from the perspective of teaching about the care than in a true academic sense. In 1997, we opened the education centre and from there on our work became not just what we did for patients but how we could bring this type of care to other health care professionals. It was important to be able to explain what palliative or hospice care is and is not. In 1999, through a confluence of events, notably the poor experience of government officials regarding the death of their parents, it was decided that palliative care should become a sub-specialty within medicine in Romania. This was quite a challenge. It was early in our development and we had very few services at that point. It was also changing the focus of medicine to some extent, and therefore we needed to encourage doctors to come and attend the courses. Having the doctors engaged was important in developing the system because the structure here places doctors as opinion leaders.

Today there are a number of services developed. Of course, most of these services are in the NGO sector and, as Romania is not a rich country, we questioned how this charitable service model could be developed throughout the country. We believed palliative care had to become part of the health system in order to reach people all over the country. We needed to engage with the legislative and financial systems to bring palliative care into mainstream health care provision. That took about seven years in all. Today palliative care is financed through the national insurance fund. We still need to shift the focus of care from hospitals towards home care because in Romania most of the people want to be at home at the end of life. We have made important steps, but palliative care is still underdeveloped. We are now facing the challenge to develop a national comprehensive palliative care system inside the present health care system. The minister of health wants a national strategy because we have regions in the country where we have no palliative care at all. In 2001, we developed minimum standards, but the real challenge is to be able to motivate people to go into this kind of work.

The compassionate practitioner

I was wondering if palliative care makes you a compassionate physician, or if you are a compassionate physician regardless of what area of practice you come from. I sometimes question whether compassion in palliative care is something inherently different, or how well compassion we show towards patients and families also translates into the way we relate with our team and with the other people in the working environment. It is sometimes difficult when you need to focus on the administrative aspects of the work and then balance that against the compassion needed to be with patients in their suffering.

I think the definition of compassion from Henri Nouwen is a good one because it is about bringing together your heart and mind in what you do for your patients. Our health care system is very biomedically orientated, and, although I am not sure this is particular to palliative care, I think compassionate work is a part of engaging as yourself, not just with your clinical skills but also with your heart, willing to enter into that sense of vulnerability. Perhaps we are exposed to greater vulnerability working with dying patients and their families compared to those working in the cure-orientated hospital system. So I think compassion is sharing that vulnerability with your patients, entering into that space and being open to enter into their suffering and not being afraid to be vulnerable. I don't know how much you can separate compassion from empathy, caring, or being a loving physician. I think they all intermingle.

I realize it may be somewhat politically incorrect to say but the Christian perspective of the definition resonates with me as a Christian myself. At the end of the day, the love that you can give to your fellow humans through caring for them is exactly what this definition evokes. Entering into and sharing that kind of suffering is as much about stripping all the pretences away and bringing your strength as a human being to the situation, inasmuch as it is about your professional capacity. It is your care as a human being, as well as your professional skill, which is important. What this person is suffering is no different to what you or I as another human being may also suffer.

So I think being compassionate is basically living your Christian faith, because I think there is very little in our medical training that really addresses what it means to be a compassionate professional. Medical training is to develop your mind but not the skills needed to enter into the world of suffering. What you can give most is the ability to care for those most vulnerable in their deepest need—the poor, the sick, those in prison, and those dying. This is deeply engrained in the Orthodox Christian doctrine. St Basil the Great modelled what we now have in the modern hospice. He took care of the sick both physically and spiritually. He cared for orphans, training them and giving them a trade. He built a town outside of the town for those who were homeless. He was really a model for this work.

The hospice movement in Romania is now moving towards a more academic development. Last year, the first chair was established and another is planned shortly. These universities will have compulsory training in palliative care in their curriculum and another five universities offer optional courses in palliative care. We also have a multidisciplinary master's in palliative care, which is also important because it helps us shape our students as health care providers towards deeper compassion and understanding of the roles of other disciplines. I think the teaching of compassion is something that can be modelled. I don't think you can learn it in the classroom through the usual methods that we use for our students. Role play with pre-given scenarios is important, obliging students to step into different shoes: the shoes of the patient, the shoes of the families, etc. The feedback from students we have taught this way was that when you get into that role, it makes you really think about the needs of that person, even if you go in with the mind of the physician.

Sometimes compassion is about the simple things that you see in your professional role but it is difficult to share when the emphasis is on professionalism and technical competence. Sometimes compassion is lost. If I work with students in the middle of their training, I can see that they have come into medicine because they want to do something good; they care about people. But by the end of the training they seem to have lost something. So I think compassion can be taught but I think it needs role modelling. It needs alternative methods of training, visual stimulation like movies, discussing images, scenarios, and stories. We need to show how much have we moved in the way we take the history of a patient, so that we don't forget the narrative history which shows the person behind the illness and helps to develop the compassionate approach.

I can offer two examples to demonstrate this. I remember we had a homeless man who was dying. We found a very distant relative and we were able to negotiate a family reunion. So this woman was there alongside the staff, sitting with the patient who was actually dying. Even though they were distantly related, she was sitting there like she had known him forever, and together with the other health care professionals, they were engaging with this man who was very gently dying. We had two emergency doctors learning about palliative care who witnessed this and they said, "This is how we should be able to provide this care, even in an emergency room. This is how every human being should be allowed to die." I think what they witnessed from that very distant family member was real compassion, almost as a stranger, distant in terms of relationship but not distant as a human being showing compassion for another person, and that was a lesson we couldn't have taught them in a classroom.

I also remember a patient with lung cancer who had a pleural infection that they had failed to drain successfully. I was with a postgraduate medical student and I remember it was terribly hard; everybody was sitting around and basically acknowledged he was dying. He was in a lot of pain but he needed to be washed. So I gave him something for the pain and I began to wash him. They couldn't believe the doctor was going to do this, but I said, 'This is what you need most at the moment.' His elderly mother was sitting there and crying and she helped me to wash him. For me, this really was entering into that place of suffering. When he was clean and peaceful, everybody was still crying and thanking me for what we did there. It was far from the role of a doctor but the student said to me, 'This is really what he needed.' This is something that remains with the people that we are training that this is something that is very difficult to put in a classroom. So that is why I am thinking that modelling—for our students, for our doctors, whomever we train—is so very important.

A case exemplar

I recall a young woman with pancreatic cancer who was very close to her little daughter, but they were a dysfunctional family. Her husband, her mother, and her mother-in-law seemed to be very cold people, and for our Latin culture this is not normal. It was as if the patient was part of the furniture. She just sat there and the conversations were very difficult. And this little girl, about four years old, was around her mother and witnessing all of this. When I went out, she took my hand and was pointing to her toys. I was sitting and playing with her and she started to talk about her kitten that had died. She asked me if that kitten would go to heaven; what would happen to that little kitten? It was so moving. And you felt that in that moment what could you do? I just sat with her, hugged her, and talked to her. At that time, we did not have social workers or psychologists on our team. Looking back at it now from the viewpoint of compassion, being with people is as important as the things we do for them. The child needed to talk about what was happening and the family was not prepared to do that. She had no other outlet. I do wonder if it was enough just to be there for that child. Was it enough in the long term to prevent that child from growing into an adult without overt traumas from early childhood? Maybe my presence with that child may have opened doors that she couldn't open anywhere else. It was clear the mother was able to talk to her child; they were always together and there was a very close link, but sometimes I am conscious how little we have available in terms of support systems for people beyond medicine.

Fostering sustainable compassion

I think this is a very challenging question. I remember the first time I attended a conference in the United States. I was very familiar with the British model and found myself wondering if developing palliative care into a kind of self-standing speciality that was being proposed risked losing the kind of initial vision that Cicely Saunders wanted of hospice and palliative care.

My feeling today is that if we try to align with other disciplines and start to speak the same language as they speak, that can only be to the benefit of palliative care. There is always a risk that we might lose the kindness, the holistic approach to compassionate aspects of care. In Romania, sometimes people say, 'Ah, you are those people who like the emotional part of the care and that takes time.' But I think this is the most valuable thing that palliative care has to offer. I remember one Swiss physician came here and he said, 'If you would help a surgeon take a gall bladder out in five minutes, he would say, Are you crazy?' So maybe if you are a palliative care physician and someone says, 'Get the patient ready in five minutes', it is equally crazy. In order for me to be able to offer the care that I want, show the compassion I want, and be present in a holistic way, I need time also.

I think if we are not careful we might lose the essence of palliative care. It would be very sad because this is the message that palliative care can be enforced for the other disciplines. My hope was when we started to put palliative care into the university curriculum, we would catch students in their younger years and try to really stretch that compassion, understand their motivation, and develop their humanistic side to match what they brought to the medical field. Compassion should be enhanced, not erased, by their training.

I was fortunate to be able to go to the San Diego Hospice to act as a mentor in a palliative care leadership programme. This programme looked at how we can develop leaders from all over the world, because in hospice care, we often develop services where a structured system does not exist, thus leadership is extremely important. San Diego wanted to bring in regional mentors to support future leaders so that they would better understand the local challenges in those systems. I became one of the mentors for Eastern Europe in this programme. I think such leadership programmes can embed the concept of compassion within practice.

I think the ideal of compassion is best transmitted in the way we work. It is not just being a compassionate physician. It is about being a compassionate person and this was visible in our working with authorities to change the legislation to establish palliative care. Whilst trying to understand the legislators' perspective, we always worked from the same model, presenting the stories of the patients and what motivated you to care for them in a compassionate way. Sometimes you felt these were rigid, bureaucratic people representing written regulations and the law, but behind that person, you found the core of a compassionate human being. That is a very good way of reaching out. People asked us in what way palliative care could be good for society. Compassion is about the kind of love that you have for another human being. These are, in a way, almost equal when you reflect on it.

Commentary

In *The Four Loves*, C.S. Lewis (2011) notes that 'to love at all is to be vulnerable. Love anything and your heart will be wrung and possibly broken' (p. 169). The impact of love in the practice and context of palliative medicine is shared here by Daniela Mosoiu and is perhaps a concept that most clinicians would feel somewhat uncomfortable with. The professional rapport expected of the health care professional would seem to be contrary to the personal and emotive nature of love. However, love and compassion share a close link, and that link may be that to love means that you are destined to suffer, as Lewis describes.

The idea of 'compassionate love' (Fehr, Sprecher, & Underwood 2008) has now become the basis of a growing body of research, notably through the work of the Fetzer Institute (http://www.fetzer.org). Work at end of life within this resource includes studies into the impact of capital punishment and nurse witness to forgiveness at life end. The term compassionate love derives from the work of these authors as a compromise to the global understanding of love across world religions. A key message from this work is that to have love for another begins with being able to love yourself. Another way to understand compassionate love is through the ideal of *loving-kindness*, one of Buddhism's four

Brahmaviharas or immeasurables, called such because they can be developed within ourselves without limit (Hangartner 2013). The four immeasurables of loving-kindness (*Mettā* or *maitri*), compassion (*Karuna*), joy (*Mudita*), and equanimity (*Upseka*) are always described together because understanding is strengthened by their interrelationship.

We often associate the concept of loving-kindness with Buddhist world views, but it is also noted in both Christian and Jewish text (חֶסֶד, sometimes translated as *Chesed*), and arises from a belief in the unconditional love of God for his people. Loving-kindness is approached at two levels. In the case example presented here, feeling deeply moved by the situation and wanting to make a difference for this little girl is only the beginning. As a doctor, the right response is to find the best way possible to address the problem—by sitting and listening to the meaning behind the story of the kitten. This brings insight that can lead to the relief of suffering for the child.

Another important element of this case is the idea of non-abandonment. Quill and Cassel (1995) described non-abandonment as a core expectation of the practice of a physician. In effect, whatever happens, the person being cared for will not suffer alone. They note that 'there is a world of difference between facing an uncertain future alone and facing it with a committed, caring, knowledgeable partner who will not shy away from difficult decisions when the path is unclear' (p. 368). Reaching out to the stranger in need (see the case of the homeless man described here) reflects the Christian archetype of the Good Samaritan. This is the response of compassionate love. We cannot prevent the impact of love on our hearts, but we can use it to respond in a truly compassionate way to our patients as well as ourselves.

Reflections for practice

♦ Consider the concept of love. How might it impact your practice as a palliative health care professional?

♦ What are the consequences of adopting the principle of non-abandonment for palliative care practitioners?

♦ What practices can you develop to sustain yourself through loving-kindness?

Further reading

Fehr B, Sprecher S, Underwood LG (eds.) (2008) The science of compassionate love: theory, research, and applications. Malden, MA: Wiley-Blackwell.

Hangartner D (2013) Human suffering and the four immeasurables: a Buddhist perspective on compassion. In T Singer, M Boltz (eds) Compassion: bridging practice and science. Munich: Max Planck Society. Chap. 8.

Lewis CS (2011) Surprised by joy/the four loves. London: Houghton Mifflin Harcourt.

Post SG, Underwood LG, Schloss JP, Hurlbut WB (eds.) (2002) Altruism and altruistic love: science, philosophy, and religion in dialogue. New York: Oxford University Press.

Quill TE, Cassel CK (1995) Nonabandonment: a central obligation for physicians. Annals of Journal of Medicine, **122**(5), 368–374.

The practice of loving-kindness (Mettā): as taught by the Buddha in the Pali Canon (comp. and transl. Ñ Thera) (2013) Access to insight (legacy ed.), 30 November.

Chapter 19

Irene Renzenbrink—
Compassionate organizations

Irene Renzenbrink is an Australian social worker who has been involved in the development of palliative care and bereavement support services in Australia since the late 1970s. She is listed in the *Who's Who* of Australian women and a member of the international work group on death, dying, and bereavement.

For over 30 years Irene has had a particular interest in the complex organizational, professional, and personal variables involved in burnout, compassion fatigue, and related phenomena. In recent years Irene has added art therapy and expressive arts therapies to her repertoire of skills, and continues to teach, write, and conduct research in the area of palliative care.

She is associate editor of the journal *Illness, Crisis and Loss* and editor of *Caregiver Stress and Staff Support in Illness, Dying and Bereavement* (Oxford University Press, 2010).

Foundations in palliative and end-of-life care

I was involved in the very first modern hospice programme in Australia, before hospice care became known as palliative care. We had the same difficulties as the Canadians about the word *hospice*. In the 1980s the term *palliative care* began to be used more widely and the word *hospice* was reserved by the religious orders to describe the more traditional free-standing hospices. I became a social worker in the early 70s and my first jobs were in cancer wards in large public hospitals. We had a pavilion-style hospital in Sydney which was just horrific. Rows and rows of patients, very much like the Florence Nightingale era. As a brand new social worker, I was assigned to a surgical tracheostomy ward. It wasn't even called an oncology ward. I had to place patients in nursing homes to die. They were closer to death than they thought. It was a terrible introduction to social work in health care. I think I learnt about compassion through the lack of it. I felt completely unsupported.

I became involved in the Melbourne City Mission Hospice which was really the first Australian programme established in the late 1970s, with funding from the Australian government and the Kellogg Foundation in the United States.

We had a Churchill fellow, Katherine Kingsbury, who went overseas and brought back the message of hospice and palliative care, and so away we went with high hopes and a reforming zeal. It got us into a lot of trouble with the medical establishment—a familiar story in many places. I started to read about the hospice movement and discovered what was happening at St Christopher's Hospice in London. It was the first example of compassionate care—patient-centred, a whole-person approach, caring for the staff, caring for the bereaved. This was music to my ears. I was a disillusioned medical social worker by then and saw this is a social reform movement that I wanted to be part of. I thought, 'This is the way forward!' This is where I can be myself and I won't have to become an insensitive sort of person in order to survive. I don't think the terms *burnout* or *compassion fatigue* were even used in those years. Charles Figley's work on compassion fatigue came later.

The first hospice programme in Melbourne had a major crisis when the medical director sacked the director of nursing. Half the staff resigned, including myself, and it was terribly disillusioning. This was only six weeks after we had admitted the first patient. The politics just became overwhelming and difficult. A few years later I went to work in another hospice. I worked in both programmes—home- and hospital-based—so I have quite a wide experience. I also spent seven years working in the funeral industry where I developed my community development skills and set up lot of bereavement support programmes. It was not an ideal base because people are nervous about funeral directors who represent our worst fears and anxieties about death. At the time they were the ones prepared to put in the resources, so ironically I found a corporate avenue for compassionate community-based care for the bereaved.

The compassionate practitioner

I think a compassionate practitioner is someone who is well trained and has enough life experience not to be thrown by difficult situations. I like the Henri Nouwen quotation about entering into places of pain, sharing in brokenness, especially brokenness. I am fascinated by the experience of fragmentation. People often say, 'I am falling apart', 'I am shattered', or 'I am heart-broken.' That language reflects their confusion and anguish. Family members often draw people into conversations such as 'What did the doctor say?' 'Has the nurse been around with that injection?' It's all about the body. So I think a compassionate response would tune into where people are, and if there is anxiety and fear, or that sense of brokenness, we need to be receptive to the symbolic language that patients use. It does not always have to be deep and meaningful; it can be playful and creative.

I think expressive arts therapies have enormous value and potential. Expressive arts therapies blend various modalities—visual art, music, creative writing, poetry—you might use all of them. I think they also have a potential use in staff support. I had staff dropping in to my studio space in the palliative care unit. They seemed to enjoy the opportunity to play with art materials and share their stories. This kind of activity takes people into an imaginary realm that is quite nourishing. They go back to the patients feeling renewed, with more energy. Art therapy represents an empowering approach for patients, families, and staff. It is based on the concept of *poesis*, the ancient Greek word for making or shaping. Poetry derives from the same word. When you work with clay, art materials, collage, perhaps you are figuratively putting yourself together again. It is quite a mysterious process.

I call on my artistic knowing as a practitioner—I might be writing poetry or doing some of my own art-making in response to the images that patients, family members, and staff create. I find it very nourishing to the spirit and I have seen this in patients, even when they feel frail and ill with this tremendous loss of bodily capacity. They just seem to feel a stronger sense of 'I am able, I can still do this.' It's not so much about exhibiting art; it is more the therapeutic relationship and process that is important in that context.

I have come across the concept of impingement by Donald Winnicott, better known for his work on transitional objects and child development. The world seems to crowd in on all of us, because we are not just palliative care practitioners, we are members of societies, members of families. It's because of the way the news is broken in our homes through radio, TV, and newspapers. I remember hearing today of an earthquake in the Philippines, people being buried alive. If you are compassionate you will be sensitive to wider issues in society. I feel compassion when I hear this terrible story about the Philippines, but if that happened here now in my own city, it would have an even deeper impact and I might feel compassion in a different way. If you are a compassionate human being I am not sure how you distinguish between the suffering at home and suffering in other places; some of us have family members in other parts of the world, too. This awareness can put us into overload at times.

It seems to me there was a lot of reassurance for staff when we had really good bereavement support programmes after the death—because they didn't have to go on carrying patients emotionally, they didn't carry the family. It was a relief that there was a new team of colleagues looking after the bereaved, and that there was still a link with the hospice. In the current economic climate, bereavement care seems to be the first thing to go. A lot of support programmes are out in the community. You might never see a person that you've helped again and yet you may have had the most profound encounters with them at the patient's bedside. After the patient has died, the contact ends. There is no continuity, no resolution for the staff. So a compassionate practitioner is one who gives people the time that they need. There can be misunderstandings between practitioners about their roles, and I think that can erode or devalue compassion.

Compassion borders on spirituality and innate personal qualities. It has to be nurtured, encouraged, modelled. It is the place where our vulnerability meets the patient's vulnerability. Caregivers are always very reluctant to expose vulnerability. When you see people in grief support sharing some of the deepest, most wounded part of themselves, they allow themselves to be open and vulnerable. As caregivers we need to match people in that vulnerability to some extent and model an authentic way of caring for others.

I used to be accused of being too thin-skinned. I thought, Well, how could I not be if I'm going to be effective in this work? I do need to be thin-skinned but I also need to find some balance in my workload. We had one manager who said everyone in the team needed to do something for their soul. So we all had to have a creative project of something we loved to balance the less appealing work. I have probably seen more vulnerability in bereavement care because that is when the defences are down. We need to allow the grief to flow, and hear the stories, however painful. I think grief support preserves that capacity to attach and be compassionate with other people. If nobody supports you when you are heartbroken, I think you can develop a hardened heart. If you are comforted and supported, you, in turn, will have the ability to comfort and support someone else. Grief and bereavement is one of the most important contributions of the hospice movement to society because it helps to preserve the capacity for love and attachment.

A case exemplar

The case that comes to mind is one where my compassion was not rewarded. It was actually judged quite harshly because of the time it took to help a patient find a suitable home. We had a slow-stream rehabilitation ward in the hospice. An Italian man in his 90s was brought into the hospice with a broken ankle. He had tripped on the tram line and fallen. He was very angry, frustrated, and wanted to sue the city of Melbourne. Actually he wanted to sue everyone! He was a rather difficult person to manage. Very volatile, very dramatic. He'd say, 'Give me a gun and I will shoot myself' and 'Put me in a box and put me in the ground.' The nurses were really stretched, so their compassion was also stretched to the limit and they wanted him out.

As soon as he was well enough to be discharged, it was my job as a social worker to find a place for him to live. I always have difficulty with that term, *placement*—the placement of people as objects. We looked at many different homes. He was in a wheelchair and I had a big station wagon, so I put the wheelchair in the back of the car and off we went. I was so appalled by the standard of some of these homes for the elderly—we call them special accommodation houses—there was nothing special about them. There would be one teaspoon of jam sitting on a plate that was each resident's allowance for the jam they could put on toast in the morning. It was very bleak.

My client had lived in a rooming house in the middle of a very vibrant area of Melbourne. He had all his favourite haunts. He wanted to be in an area that he knew, felt comfortable in. There were not a lot of places to choose from, so it took me a long time to find a suitable home for him. We kept going out on these excursions, and of course there were other patients needing care and placement, and meetings to attend. I think they all thought I was terribly involved emotionally because I was just taking too long over this. In supervision sessions I would be asked, 'Who did he remind me of? Did I think he was my grandfather?' I was so aware of the pressure to conform to a timetable, to empty that bed. I was torn between the institution's demands and the old man's needs as a human being. My own compassionate response was to give him all the time that he needed to choose a new home.

One day we were driving along in the rain when we saw a home that he recognized. It turned out to be the home of an old friend from a village in Italy. The friend had died, but his daughter still lived there. In the hallway there was a magnificent portrait of the daughter as a young woman, and who was the painter but my patient. He had won art competitions and had exhibited his work. He was a very gifted artist but everyone in the hospice thought he was just a nuisance. We had literally discovered hidden treasure. The friend's daughter embraced him and invited us in. While we were there, she phoned the man's nephew in Italy. They had lost contact. It was really a wonderful outcome for him. He had a family. He had a friend. He finally found a place that he liked—a hostel with mostly elderly women—he was such a charming fellow. He was loved and brought into the fold until he died.

I paid the price because I was seen as incompetent, was reprimanded by the senior social worker and the medical director, who both said that we cannot provide this kind of luxurious Rolls-Royce service. I found that devastating. It was terribly unfair. They were not thanking me for doing a good job at all. I knew I had done a good job; I knew that our man was happy where he settled. It was an extraordinary meeting that day, an extraordinary discovery to find a family member and a friend. None of that was recognized. If you are putting heart-and-soul energy into this work, and not valued you become disillusioned, and eventually I left. It wasn't just that incident. I was able to do a lot of good work there and felt some respect from my colleagues but not from superiors. I did not enjoy working in a place where there was no recognition. There has to be reciprocity. Sometimes the rhetoric does not match the reality. So that was my lesson about compassion.

Fostering sustainable compassion

As I see it, compassion is always under threat, particularly when resources are scarce, or when members of the multidisciplinary team are inclined to be competitive with one another. I am aware from Balfour Mount's writings of setting up the palliative care unit in Montreal that he really had to work at building a caring team, an effective team that would collaborate and not compete. It has a lot to do with maturity and self-awareness and, I would add, humility. There are very strong individuals and egos in hospice care and tensions can arise.

When Beverley Raphael gave a lecture at an International Grief and Bereavement Conference in Australia in 1991, she spoke about the need to 'develop and preserve' compassion, and that had me thinking that compassion isn't something innate. To some extent compassion is developed in our education and training as health care professionals. It is one of the values we are urged to adopt. Mary Vachon's studies were enlightening and helped me understand that compassion can be lost unless you keep working at it through professional development and team building. Unless it is preserved it will be eroded and lost. You can lose it very easily. Unfortunately it has been my negative experiences in palliative care that have prompted my interest in staff support and staff stress. The economic imperative has become increasingly important in hospice and palliative care. Hospices today are more accountable for the donations and government funding they receive. Technology has changed a lot of the practices. New data systems require specialist training. At times it seems that staff are besieged by the demands of paperwork. Social workers have complained to me about the relentlessness of e-mail referrals. So the sheer volume of the work, the lack of time to get to know each other as members of the team, the pressure to deliver services promptly, is all difficult. I think it ultimately boils down to stress over the nature of the work and death anxiety related to the witnessing of suffering over and over again. It's probably a combination of all these things.

Mary Vachon mentions a number of important variables related to individual personalities, the organization itself, and the nature of terminal illness, especially complex symptoms which cannot be managed as quickly as everyone would like. I have seen leaders who were not trained in health care professions become administrators of these services. They really don't understand the suffering. I have often seen a gap between mission statements on the wall and what is actually happening in practice. We need enlightened, clinically orientated leaders who are not afraid to validate staff suffering. The fact that staff do experience suffering should not be seen as a blot on the organization's reputation.

Managers should recognize that staff stress and grief is normal and not a sign of weakness or self-indulgence. A palliative care social worker once said to me, 'There is nowhere for the grief to go.' She and her colleagues were dismayed about a new agency policy directive. They were being asked to see newly diagnosed oncology patients. However, patients going through treatment for cancer expecting to survive have very different needs from those who are dying. Staff felt torn between these two groups of clients. Now, palliative care is moving more into the aged care sector. I fear that hospice staff are losing their specialist edge when they are expected to do so much. The stuttering dying trajectory of frail aged patients has been described by Mercedes Bern Klug as ambiguous dying. Staff may have much longer attachments with patients and families. Compassion that needs to be sustained over time is an issue. So I think being a palliative care practitioner in today's climate is very hard.

Technology has helped everyone to be much faster and more efficient but I do think we are losing something. Medical consultations where the doctor is staring at the computer screen instead of really attending to the patient are often reported by people who enter palliative care from the acute care system. Rushing about with a pager and responding to every single e-mail and every single request is so stressful. I remember working with a pager and I'd feel haunted by that sound. It was just so insistent and immediate.

Moving forward, it is interesting to see what Robin Youngson is achieving in New Zealand, forming a whole counter-revolution of compassionate health care training (Youngson 2012). I think the fact that he is a doctor is giving that effort greater legitimacy. It goes back to Cicely Saunders being told that she had to study medicine because she would not be taken seriously otherwise. The Boston Schwartz Center is another brilliant example of how you can formalize compassionate care. I think it has to be named as a goal, and dedicated resources are needed if the effort to educate and train people is to succeed. As social work students in the late 60s, early 70s, we were taught to practise 'controlled emotional involvement' and 'detached concern'. I remember weeping in the toilets in the oncology unit and it was actually a priest who supported me when one of the patients I had a long involvement with died. So you don't always find it where you think you should—your line manager, supervisor, or professional colleague. You might find it outside. But not amongst the patients. There is a danger of getting emotionally involved with patients because your needs are not being met anywhere else so you might find the patients are really looking after you and helping you feel good. Then they die and you are abandoned again.

I think we can sustain compassion because there is a hunger for a kinder approach. People are searching for another way of working with people. The rising interest in spirituality in palliative care is putting compassion back on the agenda. It seems to be the more natural vehicle for exploring big questions about meaning and suffering. Questions are raised about how we look after ourselves and where we draw our strength from. We can't be compassionate unless we have that nourishment of spirit. The huge emphasis on measurement and evidence-based practice is a sort of double-edged sword. You gain legitimacy to be able to argue for funding and resources based on evidence, but it risks denying other more subtle ways of knowing.

Trying to measure compassion is like trying to measure love. How do you smile or touch a person's hand in a caring way? It is not quantifiable. So if we could believe that other ways of knowing are valuable, I think there is definitely hope for the future. Staff support is integral to quality patient care. It is a quality assurance issue. We have to invest in staff to get the best outcomes. I think we need to send a message to the leaders and managers in hospice and palliative care about being more compassionate towards staff and to stop denying the complexity of their experiences of caring. Validate their suffering; allow grief to be expressed. Provide supervision, education and training, and time out when needed. Let's be more courageous about facing the dark side of caring. Then we will learn a lot more about compassion.

Commentary

Robin Youngson, whom Irene Renzenbrink cites, is an excellent example of compassion in action. As a doctor in the UK, his experience of the poor hospital care of his daughter underpinned his desire to challenge health care organizations to place compassion as the essence of their daily clinical practice, decision-making, and outcome measurement. Irene's experience also shows the impact that organizations can have on the compassionate response of the individual health practitioner and the need for such organizations to embrace a more staff-centred approach to their mission and vision. The theologian Ilia Delio (2005) reflects, 'There is a relationship between soul and space which is being lost and this loss, I believe, is at the heart of our ecological and economic crises' (p. 25). He concludes that the soul needs space to be enabled to grow. Health care organizations hold some responsibility in ensuring that the soul of the organization—ostensibly the staff as its greatest asset—is carefully nurtured. Martin Heidegger (2010) argued that we seek home as a place of safety and security because it protects us from the threat of death. In the case offered by Irene Renzenbrink, the search for the right place for the elderly client to live and die

demonstrates how a compassionate response is sometimes an intuitive knowing of the right thing to do, even if there are adverse consequences. The gap
between soul and space is not something alien to palliative care practitioners.
We often consider this in the debate between 'doing for' and 'being with'.
Leathard (2004) offers a contemporary Thomistic (i.e. from the perspective of
the medieval Catholic theologian, Thomas Aquinas) view of health and healing
and argues that an understanding of relationship ('relationality') is central to
the nature of being (p. 113). Understanding the relationship between organizations and their employees, the personal and political agendas that impact on
clinical comportment, and the external factors which impact on the delivery of
palliative and end-of-life care are integral to developing a compassionate service situated in mutual respect and shared governance.

Reflections for practice

♦ How is the concept of compassion envisioned in your organization?

♦ To what extent do the mission and values of your organization use the term
  compassion to describe its work?

♦ Is there a mismatch between reality and rhetoric, as Irene Renzenbrink
  suggests?

♦ If so, how can or should you address that as a health care practitioner?

Further reading

Bern-Klug M (2004) The ambiguous dying syndrome. Health and Social Work, **29**(1),
    35–65.

Delio I (2005) Compassion: living in the spirit of St Francis. Cincinnati, OH: Franciscan
    Media.

Heidegger M (2010) Being and time (rev. ed. of the Stambaugh transl.). SUNY series in
    contemporary continental philosophy. Albany, NY: SUNY Press.

Leathard HL The nature of being: a Thomistic perspective related to health and healing.
    Spirituality and Health International, **5**(2), 107–115.

Renzenbrink I (ed.) (2011) Caregiver stress and staff support in illness, dying and bereave-
    ment. Oxford: Oxford University Press.

Youngson R (2012) Time to care: how to love your patients and your job. Raglan, NZ:
    Rebelheart.

Chapter 20

Mary Vachon—The light and the shadow

Mary Vachon is a nurse, clinical sociologist, psychotherapist, researcher, educator, and cancer survivor. She is currently a consultant and psychotherapist in private practice, professor in the Department of Psychiatry and Dalla Lana School of Public Health at the University of Toronto, and clinical consultant at Wellspring.

She is a graduate of the Massachusetts General Hospital School of Nursing from which she received an alumnae achievement award in 1998. She received her bachelor of science degree from Boston University, her master of arts in sociology from the University of Toronto, and her PhD from York University, Toronto.

She has published over 170 scientific articles and book chapters on issues related to bereavement, occupational stress in health care professionals, cancer survivorship, family stress dealing with life-threatening illness, spirituality, and palliative care. On the same wide range of topics, Dr Vachon has delivered over 1,600 lectures around the world.

She is the recipient of many awards, including the Mara Morgenson Flaherty lectureship of the Oncology Nursing Society for excellence in psychosocial oncology in 1985; the Dorothy Ley Award for excellence in palliative care from the Ontario Palliative Care Association in 1997; the National (US) Hospice and Palliative Care Organization's 2001 distinguished researcher award, and, in 2008, the lifetime achievement award from the *International Journal of Palliative Nursing*.

Foundations in palliative and end-of-life care

I grew up with a number of deaths. My first memory is the day after my brother Richard was killed. We were in a car accident. I was three and he was eight weeks. I am the eldest and he was the fourth of four children we had in the family at that point; the family grew to 13. My mother was Irish Catholic and my father was Lithuanian so perhaps not surprising!

There was chronic grief in my family, particularly my father. Both of his parents had died by the time he was 17—his father when he was 12 and his mother when he was 17. He witnessed her death giving birth to his stepsister, who was then put into an orphanage. My father never really grieved his parents' deaths. We were in the process of adopting his sister and were coming back from the orphanage when the accident occurred. The Protestant neighbours were very critical that my parents were having so many kids. They said my mother had implied he had not wanted this child and my father was accused of manslaughter. My father's stepbrother was also killed when he was 22. There was a lot of drama and death in my childhood.

The Catholic religion was an integral part of my upbringing. When I was 17, I got a scholarship to nursing school at Massachusetts General Hospital (MGH). I was interviewed by the newspaper and they asked why I wanted to be a nurse. I said, 'I thought it was a Catholic woman's duty to serve mankind.' That, in fact, is what my life has been. I have travelled the world, I have had a very interesting, exciting career, but it has been a life of service.

When I was a third-year student at MGH during my ICU experience, a first-year student came to me and said, 'Mrs X was crying, she got all upset because she got faeces on her hands', and asked what should she do. I said, 'I don't know, I am going to a lecture about grief, go back and talk to her and try to figure out what is going on.' So I went to listen to this lecture on the work of Erich Lindemann who was still at MGH. I learnt all about anticipatory grief, delayed grief, chronic grief.

When I went back the next day, Mrs X was on cardiac precautions but did not know why. She said, 'They think that I have had a heart attack, but I don't think that.' I said, 'Well, yesterday I learnt all about grief. When you came in for this endarterectomy'—which was very big surgery at that point—'you might have died. You did not go through any anticipatory grief, thinking you might die. Maybe now as you are going to be discharged, you are, in fact, going through that grief.' It turned out that 16 years ago to that day, her husband had been coming back from the Korean war and she realized she no longer loved him. The boat docked in Boston Harbour and he had a heart attack and died. Now she was going through this whole experience of delayed grief and had this 'pseudo' heart attack.

I told my nursing instructor, 'I am going to go into psychiatric nursing to learn how to talk to people. If you talk to them, you find out what you think they are here for is not really the whole root of their problem.' l graduated from MGH, got my degree from Boston University, did psychiatry, and taught neurology and psychiatric nursing at MGH. In 1969, my husband and I left for Canada as Vietnam War draft dodgers. My husband had been in a Trappist monastery and did not feel this was a just war. He was accepted at the University of Toronto for graduate school and we left Massachusetts, not knowing if we would ever be able to return to the United States, but feeling this was an ethical decision we had to make.

Soon after we moved to Canada we became friendly with a couple at church. One day she wasn't at church. She was in the hospital with a bleeding nose that wouldn't stop. I said to my husband that I suspected there was a major problem and this family was going to need help, so we should get close to them. We made a calculated decision to do so. It turned out that when she was pregnant with her fourth child she had developed melanoma. The disease had now metastasized. There was little that could be done in those days. I spoke to Dr Stan Freeman, the psychiatrist with whom I was working, and asked how I could be helpful to this 37-year-old with four kids who was going to die. He said if I was interested in that sort of thing I should go to the Princess Margaret Hospital (the local cancer hospital) because they were looking for someone to work with the nurses about their feelings around dying patients. This was before there was any real thought of palliative care. A patient had died after one of the first bone marrow transplants. The nurses were upset because the doctors were not supporting them and went to one of the doctors to complain, finding him crying in his own office. So, in 1970, my colleagues and I started doing research into the stress that the nurses and physicians were experiencing. More than 40 years later, the stress is the same, and that is where compassion becomes extremely important. We need to train staff to have compassion for themselves and for those for whom they care. I think this is where we need to focus at least some of our efforts.

At the time I sought out Dr Freeman's advice, he was in process of developing the Social and Community Psychiatry Department of the Clarke Institute of Psychiatry (now the Centre for Addiction and Mental Health). I became a member of the department. The purpose of the unit was to research the concepts of Dr Gerald Caplan on the primary, secondary, and tertiary prevention of mental illness and develop interventions to measure whether intervention would make a difference. When we went to Princess Margaret Hospital we developed an intervention for the nurses and physicians and measured its efficacy. I then suggested doing an intervention with dying persons and their family members to see if we could make a difference. It was felt this would be too complicated, so we applied for funding for two studies; an intervention with women with breast cancer and an intervention with newly widowed women.

We won the research grants and simultaneously conducted the three studies. It was a very exciting time. In my 20s, I became a principal investigator on a large grant regarding bereavement intervention using a widow-to-widow programme, based on the work of Phyllis R. Silverman. I remember the big envelope that came and realizing that when I open this envelope my life is going to change.

After that, my colleague Dr Alan Lyall met Dr Balfour Mount at a meeting. Dr Mount was about to open the Palliative Care Unit at the Royal Victoria Hospital (RVH) in Montreal and suggested we come and study the stress of staff at the RVH. We went before the unit opened and we went every three months for the first two years that they were in existence. That is really how I got involved in palliative care. When I turned 60, I received my full professorship in the Department of Psychiatry. When I was doing my professorial address, the person introducing me said I was 'a clinician scientist and an expert in knowledge transfer' before the days that became a recognized concept. I was doing the research and clinical work at the same time. The clinical work always informed the research.

The compassionate practitioner

The traditional Buddhist definition of compassion involves recognizing that the other person is suffering and wanting to alleviate that suffering. I like the work of Nouwen, but when I saw the definition, I sense it is also talking about blurred boundaries. If you look at empathy as walking in the other person's shoes, this definition is a bit like empathy. The Nouwen definition does not seem to recognize that I too am suffering. In some ways, as wonderful as this definition is, you can be lost in it—one could feel when one is being compassionate you are immersed in it. So, I think we need to go beyond it.

Many of us go into this work because we had some early childhood experiences. If we have not identified our own issues and learned to separate them from what belongs to 'the other' we can over-identify. My meditation teacher uses the analogy of knots. All of our life experiences are like knots. If we don't untie our own knots when trying to 'become clear and transparent human beings on the road to enlightenment', others can hook into our knots. If we identify too strongly with the pain of the other, in part because of some unresolved issues of our own, we are unable to do anything to help them.

Compassion is about a sense of coherence—meaning that sense of power being appropriately vested. I am helped in the work that I do with a deep belief system which does not have the answers to anything, recognizes that life is a mystery and that there is some meaning in the suffering that I don't understand, and that is OK.

One of the things that is helpful to me from a Christian perspective is the metaphor of the mystical body of Christ, whereby the heart beats for the brain, the lungs, the legs, everything. Everything is connected, so for me being a part of the mystical body of Christ, whatever tiny little bit I am, I need to do my part.

I learned about this 'connection' most vividly through my experience with stage 4 non-Hodgkins lymphoma in 1996. I had many experiences with the cancer that took me to places I had never yet been and gave me insights that I had never had. One of the more unusual experiences was of feeling that I was being 'walked through' the experience of chemotherapy by 'people from the other side'. I called them my 'angels' but gradually came to recognize that I was being accompanied through my journey not only by my family members and friends who had died, but also by the people I had accompanied through their cancer journey, as well as those whose bereft relatives I had worked with. One day the priest at Mass spoke about his understanding of the Communion of Saints being reflected in the final scene of *Les Misérables* when Jean Valjean is dying and all those he had known who had died come to be with him. I came to truly understand how we are all connected and the work we do lives on.

These insights helped me with my understanding of compassion. I have learned a great deal from the work of Roshi Joan Halifax from the Upaya Zen Center who has studied this topic in detail. Her latest and very different definition describes compassion as 'the capacity to be attentive to the experience of others, to wish the best for others, and to sense what will truly serve others' (Halifax 2014). Ironically, in a time when we hear the term compassion fatigue with increasing frequency, she argues that compassion does not lead to fatigue. In fact, it can become a wellspring of resilience to allow our natural impulse to care for another to become a source of nourishment rather than depletion. Crucial to the concept of compassion is that we cannot practise compassion for others if we do not practise self-compassion. As we concluded in an article I wrote with Drs Michael Kearney, Balfour Mount, and colleagues in 2009, 'The heart first pumps blood to its self.' (p.1162)

I think I see compassion in action when people go beyond what they *need* to do. A personal example from years ago was when I had a colonoscopy without any kind of anaesthesia or analgesia. I was just screaming in pain and the nurse reached out and held my hand. That to me is compassion—reaching out and accompanying another on her journey, trying to alleviate her suffering. The next time I asked for sedation but it didn't work. I reached out for the nurse's hand, but she said I was hurting her and pulled her hand away. It was a much more isolated kind of experience.

Since my cancer experience, I have developed daily meditation practice and recite the serenity prayer and the prayer of St Francis. Daily, I set my intention to have the serenity to 'accept the things that I cannot change, the courage to change the things I can and the wisdom to know the difference', and asking to be an 'instrument'. I ground myself in these intentions before starting my day. When I don't know what to do with a client I just say, 'make me an instrument', and something comes. I think when we truly embrace compassion, we are beyond ego and recognize that we are connected with something much bigger than ourselves. This to me is part of the sense of coherence, power as 'appropriately vested'. I remember reading that people with a sense of coherence have greater enthusiasm. The root of enthusiasm is *en theos*, in God.

Sometimes we do or say something and we don't know where it comes from. Compassion links to spirit for me. I see spirit as the feminine aspect of the Godhead; it is about wisdom. I draw very heavily on the work of Hildegard von Bingen and the idea of *veriditas* and *veritas*. I strongly connect with her image of the Man in Sapphire Blue. As Matthew Fox said of this image, compassion is taking the energy of the heart chakra and putting it into the hands. He describes this man as being one whose body is in his soul, rather than one whose soul is in his body. Within the energy layers surrounding the man's body, there is an opening in the man's crown chakra. I think of it as a portal to bring in energy from the universe and release what we do not need to keep.

A couple of years ago, Roshi Joan Halifax had a grant at the Smithsonian Institute to study if compassion could be taught. She wrote a very dense but valuable article about her work at the Smithsonian for a journal I co-edited. She, like Tania Singer, talks about the difference between compassion and empathy. Recent neuroscience research shows that the ability to tune into one's own body sensations activates the same brain circuits (within the insula cortex) as those of empathy. As one tunes into one's body with meditation and becomes conscious of ourselves and others, you can see that connection through brain pattern activity. We are wired to each other. I frequently quote the Shanfelt study which showed that internal medicine residents who had some kind of self-care which included meditation and spiritual practice were more empathic with patients (Shanafelt 2005).

Halifax suggests this may be one base for the development of empathy and compassion. Self-awareness and self-compassion may prime our brains towards empathy and compassion for others. Recent research by Weng and colleagues has shown that people who did seven hours of compassion meditation training and had the highest levels of altruism were the ones who experienced the most brain changes in the inferior parietal cortex (involved in empathy) when exposed to others' suffering (Weng et al 2013).

I was thinking of a metaphor to describe the difference between empathy and compassion. The idea of *exquisite empathy* (deep sensitive empathic engagement) and *empathic strain* (the impact of being empathic on the caregiver) is evident in the very recent work of Singer and Bolz, incorporating both the breadth and depth of the science and art of compassion. My son teaches child and youth workers. He said his students define empathy as 'walking in another's shoes'. The poem 'Footprints' came to mind. I suddenly had this image that empathy can be walking in the shoes of the other person and for whatever reason those shoes may not fit you—you can have difficulties with boundaries of empathic strain because the shoes do not fit, or you can think these shoes do not fit me, and throw them away. With exquisite empathy you can walk in these shoes one way or another. Or you can walk beside the person and accompany them on their journey. It reminds me of another quotation which is commonly attributed to Albert Camus: 'Don't walk behind me; I may not lead. Don't walk in front of me; I may not follow. Just walk beside me and be my friend.'

Recent research also shows that compassion reduces physiological stress and promotes physical and emotional well-being. Singer's work with Mathieu Ricard, a meditation adept, demonstrating that using meditation, the response to empathy in the brain differs from compassion, is very exciting. This is all very new stuff but the evidence is coming.

A case exemplar

Annabelle was a 53-year-old artist, diagnosed with endometrial and later breast cancer. She used her art to help her cope with the distress. She wanted people to be witness to her art. When her physicians were not prepared to look at her art, it was as though they did not care about her. One of her paintings, reproduced in the chapter I wrote in the *Oxford Textbook of Palliative Medicine*, is of a ship on a stormy sea, with a cross on it called HMS Chemotherapy. There is a wine cork bobbing in the sea saying, 'God bless her and all who sail on her.' She felt she was the wine cork. There is a lighthouse because they were very important to her. She had a poor relationship with her parents. As a child, she developed a relationship with the 'Light', sensing it would speak to her in difficult times and tell her what good parents would be doing in the situation.

She had major problems with anxiety and attachment, and had simultaneously seen both a female and male psychiatrist who essentially served as parent figures. She had frequently self-referred to mental health institutions. Both her psychiatrists had died by the time she was diagnosed with her cancer and she was referred to me. When she was on the palliative care unit, she would scream and the staff did not really know how to handle that. At one point a chaplain, seeking to be helpful, asked, 'What do you believe in?' She clenched and pounded her fist and said, 'I believe in Mary Vachon!' This said, she was surrounded by compassionate caring professionals. She was able to establish a good relationship with her oncologist who took the time to look at her art; her radiation oncologist admired her collection of pearl necklaces, and her surgeon recognized her as the author of numerous letters to the editor of a local newspaper. At one point she felt unsafe at home and went into a senior's residence for care. I asked the clinical team if they would consider admitting her to the palliative care unit when she was initially receiving radiation treatment for her metastatic disease. This was not at a time when palliative care admission would normally be considered. Yet, they did!

One day in winter, when I did a home visit to Annabelle prior to her diagnosis of metastatic disease, she told me that she had a dream in which four angels with a hovercraft came to her, and they said, 'We are the June angels; we have come to take you to a safe place.' I said nothing to Annabelle but thought it might mean that she would die in June. There was no indication at that point that she had metastatic disease, which was confirmed shortly after. When she was later admitted to the palliative care unit, she said, 'This is the room that those angels came and took me to—so this is my safe place.'

Annabelle frequently screamed through her dying and I was growing increasingly concerned that maybe we needed to do something more to help her. I had considered asking my friend Maria, who practised Therapeutic Touch® for people with cancer, to see her. One day we were at a meditation class together. I had not mentioned Annabelle. Afterwards, my friend shared that in her meditation she had seen an image of a hovercraft with an angel. She had no idea what the image might mean. I told Maria that I was seeing someone who was having trouble dying, and I thought she could be helpful using Therapeutic Touch®. When I got home, there was a message from Annabelle's daughter to say that she had died that morning. So, one angel came to my friend to let us know that other three had taken Annabelle to the other side.

After her death, I reviewed my notes and found that I had visited her on 3 February, which for Roman Catholics is the feast of St Blaise when you have your throat blessed. The throat chakra is connected with creativity and speaking one's truth. Annabelle said to me, 'I will not be silenced the way my father was silenced.' She screamed frequently as she was dying and then died quite peacefully. She had drawn a picture of a skull with a padlock on the jaw, representing the way that her family of origin did not speak of things. The drawing is in the chapter in the *Oxford Textbook of Palliative Medicine*.

There is a photograph in my office from Annabelle of a library in an old mansion with light streaming onto the books. Annabelle called the image *The Light and the Word*. Two people who knew nothing of Annabelle's story have sat in that chair for meditation in which helpers come to aid and guide. They each had the Light as a helper. When they asked the Light what they should call it, the answer was 'Annabelle'.

I believe that through compassion, through reaching out, through being present to people and travelling with them wherever it is, whatever kind of space they are in, we recognize we are all suffering and must try to alleviate the suffering of every being. In many ways I feel that Annabelle continues to work with me in my practice.

Fostering sustainable compassion

There are issues in organizations related to the professionalization of palliative care and I do think some of this has to do with ego. I supervised a physician's doctoral thesis on this very issue which argued that there is a strategic shift today from the care *of* clients to care *for* clients.

The US author on spiritual healing Caroline Myss talks about the difference between a job, a career, and a vocation. A job puts a roof over our heads, gives us food, takes care of our basic needs. A career feeds the ego such as 'I am better than you . . . I have more publications than you.' This is something we very much see in health care. Vocation is service to the soul.

Many years ago, I wrote an article about motivation and what brought us into the field. Sometimes it was to do the 'in thing' and sometimes it was about convenience. A friend of mine refers to 'refrigerator nurses'. Are we there just to buy a new refrigerator? It is really important to know what brought us into the helping professions. Much of it can be about the unhealthy application of ego in practice. I had an experience in a previous post during my cancer illness when planning how my work should be covered if I was no longer able to see my clients. I discovered that colleagues were raising ethical concerns about my capacity to practice with clients in light of my own illness. There were a number of people who—due to ego, I believe—did not want me there. The issue of the scapegoat, which I wrote about in the early days of palliative care, continues to exist.

The whole concept of service is very important to compassion. Both Rachel Naomi Remen from Commonweal and Frank Ostaseski from the Metta Institute talk about service. When we serve, we serve with our full selves, not only with our skills, but with our *full* self, which includes our wounds and all that makes us. To do that we first need to have self-awareness and care for ourselves. The evidence shows that people who have a full and complete way of caring for themselves are more able to be present to clients. We can blame organizations for their failure to support, but I think that many health care providers come in to the field without a good sense of self, unconsciously wanting to serve their own unmet needs. If we don't get in touch with our own unmet needs outside of the work situation, we look for our clients and patients to do that. Individuals really need to take some responsibility for taking care of themselves because many simply do not. If we are serving as full and complete human beings, we are serving as an instrument, so it is not about me and my ego.

Everybody has to work too hard. In 1970, people were complaining about work overload and they still are today. The literature is beginning to indicate that maybe people in palliative care have more stress than other professional groups. Maybe this is because of an unrealistic desire to change the world, like

Weissman's concept of the palliative care martyr. Stephen Connor in his recent book in 2009 talks about the light and the shadow. He suggests the greater the light, the larger the shadow. If we are seen or indeed see ourselves as saints and angels, we cast a very big shadow, and we need to understand that shadow side of ourselves. In the early days, I talked about anger in hospice people and I said beware of the nice person, because under the nice person there is often a lot of anger and rage. We can operate with empathy but not necessarily in a compassionate way. The impact on us as caregivers, that empathic strain can lead to a distancing issue. I had a client whose husband's dying had not been good from a care perspective. When she discussed the awful care he received, he told her, 'Yes, but my record is going to look fine.' Indeed when they accessed his medical record it showed no deviation from optimal clinical practice. People wanted to placate her and thank her for sharing but they didn't want to do anything. She was supposed to be pleased that someone in authority had met with her. People get caught up with their own egos and are not really looking at what is going on.

There is a body of work developing around changing organizations from within through the introduction of mindful practices. As one example, Lise Fillion and Melanie Vachon in Quebec are basing work around the 'being with dying' programme from Roshi Joan Halifax, using meaning-centred interventions combined with mindfulness meditation. They want to validate a conceptual framework and choice of models for decision-makers based on a better understanding of work satisfaction and well-being of nurses in the field. The Registered Nurses Association of Ontario have just published a document about developing and sustaining inter-professional health care, optimizing patients, clients, organizations, and systems outcomes. They have looked at a number of sources of work stress and the evidence for each of these areas and what kind of interventions could be used. We need to consider what organizations do that keeps us from being what we can be and that may well be about specific individuals.

Sharon Salzberg suggests that 'Compassion is the trembling of our hearts in response to seeing pain or suffering' (http://www.sharonsalzberg.com). Compassion has energy of its own and is about connecting to something bigger than us, a sort of lifting up of our spirits, even if we are dealing with our own very difficult pain. I think this is tricky with the health care system, but the future is meeting people where they are on their journey. It is being present to help people such the woman in my case who did not want to die silently. To recognize it is their journey and to accompany them on their journey—it is not ours. I believe we are all instruments trying the make this world better.

Commentary

The Buddhist teacher Pema Chödrön considers that 'in order to have compassion for others, we have to have compassion for ourselves' (http://www.shambala.org). From 40 years of clinical and psychotherapeutic encounter, Mary Vachon takes us the heart of the compassion dialogue on the need to be attuned to ourselves in order to be able to attune to others in their suffering. In this chapter, she raises important questions for consideration: what brought me to the field of palliative and end-of-life care, and why? What understanding do I have of my life journey that may impact on the way I perceive and offer care? How do I see myself as a palliative care practitioner, and how am I seen by others? As she presents here, these may be important questions which, though challenging, can ultimately sustain.

The idea of light and shadow is an interesting one and well explored in the psychological and psychotherapeutic literature, particularly in the work of C.G. Jung. Anthony Storr (1983) offers an eclectic overview of the writings and reflections of Jung which is useful for a beginner looking to explore his work more deeply. For Jung, the shadow was 'the negative side of the personality, the sum of all those unpleasant qualities we like to hide' (Jung 1955/2014, vol 7: 107). In a more contemporary reflection, Paul Gilbert (2013) argues that sometimes these negative perceptions about ourselves can inhibit our ability to receive compassion. He makes a strong case for the impact of 'emotional memory' (p. 119) on how we perceive ourselves and respond to situations. Sometimes people find it hard to receive compassion because of the fear of exposure to deep emotions that have been untended for many years or because of an incident or belief from earlier life which impacts on the way life is currently viewed or lived. These fears or beliefs may present as difficulties in closeness, aggressive responses to situations, or a sense of shame, rejection, or abandonment. Annabelle's story and her need to be heard in the midst of her dying echoes these fears and warrant a deeper consideration of how the palliative care professional can respond to such need meaningfully and with purpose.

In the Irish language, the phrase *ar scáth a chéile a mhainimíd* translates as 'we live in the shadow of each other'. Our shared humanity means that we are equally exposed to these fears or beliefs in our own life; if one chooses to work with those who are facing the reality of life ending, perhaps there may be an onus on the practitioner to consider their own perspectives and motivations. There is a wealth of evidence that addressing self-compassion is one way to explore this. A starting point may be to take a self-compassion test (http://www.self-compassion.org). Rating on a scale of 1–5, higher scores on the sub-scales of Self-judgement, Isolation, and Over-identification indicate less self-compassion, while lower scores suggest greater self-compassion. Mindfulness and its positive impact on practitioner stress reduction is also well reported in the work of Singer and Bolz (2013) and in studies of specific professional groups (Fillion et al. 2013; Shanafelt et al. 2005; Cohen-Katz et al. 2004). The message here is that some practice that enables practitioners to care for themselves is personally meaningful and potentially clinically useful. If we can begin the process of being kind to ourselves, accept the shadows as they are, try to understand them and to 'untie the knots' that need to be untied in our own lives, without self-judgement or self-criticism, it opens the possibility of a compassionate response which enriches and nourishes rather than depletes the practitioner. Hopefully, that leads us all to Annabelle's Light.

Reflections for practice

- Consider the reasons which brought you into palliative and end-of-life care. If you are new to the field, what motivated you to turn to this discipline? If not, looking back on the reasons you came to palliative and end-of-life care, are they still valid today?

- In the case exemplar, Annabelle makes a clear statement about not being silenced in her dying. Are you challenged by her decision? How would you respond to it?

- Reflect on the words of Albert Camus in this chapter. How does that speak to your professional practice in palliative care?

Further reading

Chödrön P (2001) Start where you are: a guide to compassionate living. Boston: Shambala Classics.

Cohen-Katz J, Wiley D, Capuano T, Baker DM, Shapito S (2004) The effects of mindfulness-based stress reduction on nurse stress and burnout: a quantitative and qualitative study. Holistic Nursing Practice, 18(6), 302–308.

Connor SR, (2009) Hospice and palliative care: the essential guide. New York, Routledge.

Fillion L et al. (2013) To improve services and care at the end of life: understanding the impact of workplace satisfaction and well-being of nurses. Rapport R-794, Montréal, IRSST. http://www.irsst.qc.ca/-projet-vers-l-amelioration-des-services-et-des-soins-de-fin-de-vie-mieux-comprendre-l-impact-du-milieu-de-travail-sur-la-satisfaction-et-le-bien-etre-des-0099-6050.html

Fox M (2003) Illuminations of Hildegard of Bingen. Rochester, VT: Bear & Company.

Gilbert P (2013) Compassion-focused therapy: working with arising fears and resistances. In T Singer, M Bolz (eds.) Compassion: bridging practice and science. Munich: Max Planck Society. 112–131.

Halifax J (2014) G.R.A.C.E. for nurses: cultivating compassion in nurse/patient interactions. Journal of Nursing Education and Practice, 4(1), 121–128.

Jung C.J (2014) The collected works of C.G. Jung: complete digital edition, Adler G (Ed). New York, Princeton University Press.

Kearney MK, Weininger RB, Vachon MLS, Mount BM, Harrison RL (2009) Self-care of physicians caring for patients at the end of life: 'being connected . . . a key to my survival'. Journal of the American Medical Association, **301**, 1155–1164.

Registered Nurses' Association of Ontario (2013). Developing and sustaining interprofessional health care: optimizing patients/clients, organizational, and system outcomes. Toronto, ON: Registered Nurses' Association of Ontario.

Shanafelt, TD, West C, Zhao X, Novotny P, Kolars J, Habernmann T, Sloan J (2005) Relationship between increased personal well-being and enhanced empathy among internal medicine residents. Journal of General Internal Medicine, **20**(7), 559–564.

Singer T, Bolz M (eds.) (2013) Compassion: bridging practice and science. Munich: Max Planck Society.

Storr A (2013) The essential Jung: selected and introduced by Anthony Storr (reissue ed.). New York: Princeton University Press.

Weissman D (2011) Martyrs in palliative care. Journal of Palliative Medicine, **14**(12), 1278–1279.

Weng H, Fox AS, Shackman AJ, Stodola DE, Caldwell JZK, Rogers GM, Davidson RJ (2013) Compassion training alters altruism and neural responses to suffering. Psychological Science, **24**(7), 1171–1180.

Some of the authors cited in this chapter have web pages which highlight other publications and resources which may be of interest:

Sharon Salzberg: http://www.sharonsalzberg.com

Rachel Naomi Remen: http://wwwrachelremen.com

Caroline Myss: http://www.myss.com

The footprints poem can be downloaded: http://www.footprints-inthe-sand.com/index.php?page=Poem/Poem.php

The full quotation cited by Pema Chödrön at the beginning of the Commentary is available: http://www.shambhala.org/teachers/pema/tonglen1.php

The Registered Nurses' Association of Ontario's inter-professional practice guidelines are available: http://www.rnao.ca/bpg/guidelines/interprofessional team work healthcare

Chapter 21

Philip J Larkin—Conclusion: lessons from our teachers

Ways of knowing, ways of being

Rinpoche and Shlim (2006) argue that four kinds of teachers are needed to walk the path of spiritual enlightenment. These teachers provide us with, amongst other things, the sayings of enlightened beings to guide us, the shared knowledge and wisdom that they impart, and a deeper understanding of our innate nature. Here, the third type of teacher, one who is the 'symbolic teacher of experience' (p. 115), specifically exemplifies the wisdom and learning gleaned from the expert contributors who took time to consider, reflect, and respond to the question, Is compassion the essence of palliative and end-of-life care?

This chapter provides an overview of some of the core messages they proposed and the meaning that this holds for the current and future clinical practice of palliative and end-of-life care. Comprehensive rather than exhaustive, further readings of each chapter will, over time, no doubt offer closer understanding of the breadth and depth of clinical practice, the impact of compassion on both the practitioner and patient, and how we carry this practice wisdom forward into the twenty-first century. To draw conclusions from this learning, the contextual patterns of compassion exhibited in the experience of the 19 global palliative care experts are presented with reference to the original key questions asked of them:

- What does it means to be a compassionate practitioner of palliative and end-of-life care?

- How is compassion demonstrated and interpreted in practice?

- How can compassion be fostered and sustained for the next generation of practitioners?

In addition to the key readings and references offered at the end of each chapter, the questions above is linked to one specific text, the e-book 'Compassion; bridging science and practice by Tania Singer and Matthias Bolz (2013) which offers a focus to guide further study on the topic in relation to palliative and end-of-life care.

What does it mean to be a compassionate practitioner of palliative and end-of-life care?

The description of compassion by Nouwen et al. (1982) reflected a particular understanding that expressed the idea of compassion as 'to suffer with'. For the contributors, this was somewhat contentious. Although some considered that it had merit in describing the work of the palliative care practitioner in engaging with patients and families, there was a sense that it did not fully reflect the sense of being truly present to critically meaningful transitions points in people's lives, and that these moments for both patient and practitioner could be equally joyful, uplifting, and pleasurable. Therefore, compassion may warrant a slightly different, perhaps broader expression in the context of palliative and end-of-life care beyond its natural place in the discourse around suffering. Of interest, that discourse within clinical literature has focused particularly around suffering and the use of therapeutic sedation, a very tangible expression of the ideal of compassion in action from a palliative care perspective (Dumont et al. 2014; Schildmann & Schildmann 2014; Dass & Bush 1992). However, for the contributors, suffering needed to be seen in the context of wider dimensions, such as its potential to enhance relationship, connectedness, and engagement. These aspects of caring, which are equally prominent in the palliative care literature, are important to understanding the full meaning of a compassionate response to suffering for patients and families receiving palliative and end-of-life care (Hebblewhite 2014; Matthiesen et al. 2014; Penman et al. 2013).

Metaphor has a strong place in the description of the craft of palliative and end-of-life care. Images of journeying with, being present to, tending, holding, and nurturing all hold meaning in what it means to work clinically in this field (Mount 2013; Seno 2010; Sasser & Pulchalski 2010; Boston & Mount 2006). Exposure to the practice of clinicians in the Dana-Farber Cancer Institute afforded an opportunity to test emerging expressions of compassion derived from expert interviews through observing the work and listening to the language of compassion used in describing clinical encounter. Shared metaphors, such as 'looking through the person's eyes', 'walking in their shoes', and 'witnessing' appeared in the descriptions of compassionate care offered by contributors and observed in interactions between the hospital team and their patients. This would suggest that there is some global recognition amongst palliative care practitioners of the need to engage deeply with the suffering of patients and families in order to be of real service (another interesting concept which arose in the course of discussion). The growth of literature within palliative care scholarship that recognizes this is evidence of the multidimensional approach needed for compassionate practice (Kearney et al. 2009; Kearney 2009; Cassell 2009; Breitbart 2008; Mount & Kearney 2003).

However, equally important was the fact that clinical excellence was a pre-requisite for compassionate caregiving. True compassion was expressed through the highest levels of clinical practice which address the totality of symptom burden and complex need. Compassion was not an alternative to expert practice, and the idea that a compassionate clinician may not be seen as a clinically competent one was strongly rejected. Rather, compassion was viewed in terms of its strength and resilience which complemented the overall management of care (Halifax 2011; Feldman 2005; Chödrön 2001).

How is compassion demonstrated and interpreted in practice?

Contributors offered a broad discussion regarding both the art and science of compassionate care, which complemented the growth in understanding of the neuroscience and application of compassion. This included reflections on the relationship between faith and/or spiritual practice for compassionate caregiving and the way in which compassion could best be taught. This alludes to the question of whether compassion is innate or something that can be applied and so nurtured in the clinician.

The evidence (see parts 2 and 3 in Singer & Bolz 2013) indicates that we are, in some way, connected to each other, that we sense and express compassion cognitively and emotionally. There may well be an innate element to the presence of compassion in the human psyche. Contributors considered that people who come to the practice of palliative and end-of-life care (and indeed health care in general) bring a sense of compassion with them as their initial motivation to work in a caring profession. Within practice, it was proposed that although aspects of the compassion can be delivered theoretically, role modelling by the expert practitioner enabled a deeper sense of that compassionate essence to be distilled and incorporated in the delivery of practice. This was considered an important way in which the reality of palliative and end-of-life care practice could be demonstrated.

One expression of the balance between the innate and extrinsic meaningful to palliative and end-of-life care is expressed in the Talmudic phrase *qol dmamah dagah*—'the voice of fragile silence' that is also sometimes termed 'the still small voice' in Christian terms (Hechsel 1955). In effect, there is something within us which guides our appreciation of a given situation. Through listening to this voice we become attuned to our personal motivations and reactions, and thereby our clinical reasoning is imbued with the wisdom to make essentially the right decision in a given context. This may, for example, include a careful and reflective decision not to intervene clinically, and speaks to where compassion acts as a visible baseline to compassionate clinical engagement.

The question of whether faith was important in the embodiment of compassionate practice was polarized. Contributors either reported a strong influence in their life or that faith was not in any way predictive of either compassion or the stimulus for practice. Practically all recognized the spiritual roots of the hospice model of care advocated by Cicely Saunders as foundational to what became contemporary hospice and palliative care, and that it was important that this was not 'airbrushed' out of the narrative around historical development (Clark 2005). The influence of Cicely Saunders's *Watch with Me: Inspiration for a Life in Hospice Care* (2003) was particularly noted by some contributors. Indeed, the reflection back to Cicely Saunders's personal influence on many of them (through teaching, clinical practice, or at conferences) denotes the continuing firmament of that personal spiritual philosophy in service delivery today. Without doubt, the case exemplars presented in this book offer insight and wisdom of their own into the meaning of palliative care practice and where compassion lies within that. The range of personal, clinical, organizational, and holistic experiences gleaned suggest that compassion is visible in practice, can be named and demonstrated, and is a framework from which practitioners engage. With a strong foundation in its own spiritual history, the opportunity to embrace wider and different dimensions of world belief and practices can only enhance rather than diminish the quality of care to be given.

How can compassion be fostered and sustained for the next generation of practitioners?

Contributors did indicate that elements of practice were at risk of being lost as palliative care develops along its integrated health care trajectory. This was by no means universal and the benefits of integration with mainstream health care were also extolled. At this time, a watching brief by experts such as the contributors to this book may suffice to ensure that those aspects of practice which differentiate what palliative care can offer to the plan of care are neither subsumed nor diluted. Amidst the worries and concerns for what has been lost in palliative and end-of-life care expressed by some, there is a thread of hope for the future, underscored by the belief that compassion is a catalyst for choosing to work in a caring profession and our responsibility is to nurture it in those who present themselves for training.

Most contributors concluded that the selection of suitable candidates for the discipline of palliative and end-of-life care was a key factor in sustainability. The growing academic base of palliative care education through university courses and continuing practice development presented in many chapters, as well as efforts to include palliative and end-of-life care as core to undergraduate health care curricula, is to be welcomed. A caveat raised in this book is that academic excellence does not necessarily make an excellent practitioner since other elements (e.g. approach, communication, reflective capacity) are at play. Where being present to suffering, pain, and dying is the bread and butter of practice, the wise selection of candidates is important for themselves, the team, and the patients and families they work with. As contributors noted, the risk of using the clinical arena to address unmet personal needs around grief and loss and the need to identify indicators of resilience in the face of ongoing suffering, suggest that for some potential candidates, the most compassionate response may be to indicate that palliative and end-of-life care is not the best fit for them at this time in their career.

It is perhaps unfair to suggest that evidence presented of poor standards of care at end of life through, for example, the review of the Liverpool Care Pathway for Dying Patients (https://www.gov.uk/government/publications/review-of-liverpool-care-pathway-for-dying-patents) or the Francis Report (http://www.midstaffspublicinquiry.com) equate only to care that simply lacks compassion per se. Although this was a clear focus of media attention, both reports indicate a myriad of reasons, including inadequate training opportunities for practitioners and poor organizational support for implementation of care planning (Davis & Guyer 2013). Sean Morrison (2013) notes in his review of models of palliative care in the US that funding is key to the issue of how the public/private or voluntary/statutory interface works and determines how local or national services are delivered and reimbursed. This challenge translates equally to the global experience of health care and the delivery of palliative and hospice care in particular. What is needed are models of care which are responsive and not restrictive, and which allow the practitioner to use the fullest range of skills and opportunities, including the capacity to make compassionate decisions and appropriate judgements in the face of shifting goals of care. For those involved in the delivery of specialist palliative care education, our compassionate response to organizational failure is to provide evidence-based support and guidance to those who truly wish to learn and develop their expertise in this field of practice.

This book has not addressed the issue of compassion fatigue, although it was an underlying current in expert discourse; the need for self-care is clearly another issue of concern for the discipline (Sanchez-Reilly et al. 2013; Zambrano et al. 2013; Slocum-Gori et al. 2013; Melvin 2012; Showalter 2010). The importance of creating some system for personal support (for some, engagement in clinical supervision; for others, being able to step back from engagement when personal resources are low) indicated a self-awareness that proposes compassion begins with the self in order to reach out to others. The need for the system to harness the benefits of this for the delivery of service should be a focus for organizations who claim to have compassion as the base of their care philosophy. Therefore, compassion is not just about individual responses but rather how practitioners are enabled by systems to sustain and support themselves in the complex and challenging work that they do. We have a responsibility to ensure that the mission statement on the wall—many of which cite compassion as their ultimate measure of excellence—becomes a reality and not an aspiration.

Final thoughts

The late Irish poet and philosopher John O'Donohue (1956–2008) reflected on the need for compassion as a constant in our world today. Given the international conflicts and threats to health and well-being globally, it is a call for commitment in the face of crisis. O'Donohue proposed that compassion is derived from using one's heart wisely in the care of others. For me, this describes the daily practice of those who choose to work in palliative and end-of-life care. The importance of heart in the description and delineation of compassion was indicated by many contributors to this book who, it would seem, do consider compassion to be meaningful to the fullest expression of palliative and end-of-life care. Does that, therefore, make it the essence? If the essence of something is about its character and indispensable quality, then the expressions of compassion indicated in this book would propose that palliative and end-of-life care without compassion is a most unlikely occurrence. Technological advancement is a benefit of our age. Its wise and judicious use, whilst not losing sight of compassion as our key motivation, will be the challenge which the discipline will continue to debate. His Holiness the Dalai Lama (2010) argues that compassion is the genuine concern of all people. It may be the particular concern of those in palliative and end-of-life care as a means to shape clinical excellence in practice and provide a compass to guide the direction and focus of practice as we embrace the challenges of twenty-first-century health care. That is, at least, my hope.

Further reading

Boston PH, Mount BM (2006) The caregiver's perspective on existential and spiritual distress in palliative care. Journal of Pain and Symptom Management, **32**(1), 13–26.

Breitbart W (2008) Thoughts on the goals of psychosocial palliative care. Palliative and Supportive Care, **6**, 211–212.

Cassell E (2009) Suffering. In D Walsh et al. (eds.) Palliative medicine. Philadelphia: Saunders Elsevier, chapter **9**: 46–51.

Chödrön P (2001) Start where you are: a guide to compassionate living. Boston: Shambala Classics.

Clark D (2005) Cicely Saunders: selected writings, 1958–2004. Oxford: Oxford University Press.

Dalai Lama, Stril-Rever S (2010) My spiritual journey. New York: HarperCollins.

Dass R, Bush M (1992) Compassion in action: setting out on the path of service. New York: Bell Tower.

Davis C, Guyer C (2013) Integrated care pathways for dying patients—myths, misunderstandings and realities in clinical practice. European Journal of Palliative Care, 20(3), 112–119.

Dumont S et al. (2014) The use of palliative sedation: a comparison of attitudes of French-speaking physicians from Quebec and Switzerland. Palliative and Supportive Care, 14, 1–9.

Feldman C (2005) Compassion: listening to the cries of the world. Berkeley, CA: Rodmell.

Halifax J (2011) The precious necessity of compassion. Journal of Pain and Symptom Management, 41(1), 146–152.

Hebblewhite A (2014) A medical student's reflection on palliative care: managing emotional connection with patients. Palliative and Supportive Care, 27, 1–4.

Heschel AJ (1955) God in search of man. New York: Torchbooks.

Kearney M (2009) A place of healing: working with nature and soul at the end of life. New Orleans, LA: Spring Journal.

Kearney MK, Weininger RB, Vachon MLS, Mount BM, Harrison RL (2009) Self-care of physicians caring for patients at the end of life: 'being connected . . . a key to my survival'. Journal of the American Medical Association, 301, 1155–1164.

Mathiesen M, Froggatt K, Owen E, Ashton JR (2014) End-of-life conversations in care: an asset-based model for community engagement. BMJ Supportive & Palliative Care. doi 10.1136/bmjspcare-2013-000516

Melvin CS (2012) Professional compassion fatigue: what is the true cost of nurses caring for the dying? International Journal of Palliative Nursing, 18(12), 606–611.

Morrison RS (2013) Models of palliative care delivery in the United States. Current Opinion in Supportive and Palliative Care, 7(2), 201–206.

Mount B (2013) Healing, quality of life and the need for a paradigm shift in palliative care. Journal of Palliative Care, 29(1), 45–48.

Nouwen HJM, McNeill DP, Morrison DA (1982) Compassion: a reflection on the Christian life. New York: Doubleday.

O'Donohue J (2003) Divine beauty: the invisible embrace. London: Bantam.

Penman J, Oliver M, Harrington A (2013) The relational model of spiritual engagement depicted by palliative care clients and caregivers. International Journal of Nursing Practice, 19(1), 39–46.

Rinpoche CN, Shlim D (2006) Medicine and compassion: a Tibetan lama's guidance for caregivers. Somerville, MA: Wisdom Publications.

Sanchez-Reilly S, Morrison LJ, Casey E, Bernacki R, O'Neill L, Kopo J (2013) Caring for oneself to care for others: physicians and their self-care. Journal of Supportive Oncology, 11(2), 75–81.

Sasser CG, Pulchalski CM (2010) The humanistic clinician: traversing the science and art of health care. Journal of Pain and Symptom Management, 39(5), 936–940.

Saunders C (2003) Watch with me: inspiration for a life in hospice care. London: Mortal Press.

Schildman E, Schildman J (2014) Palliative sedation therapy: a systematic literature review and critical appraisal of available guidance on motivation and decision-making. Journal of Palliative Medicine, 17(5), 601–611.

Seno VL (2010) Being-with dying: authenticity in end-of-life encounters. American Journal of Hospice and Palliative Medicine, 27(6), 377–386.

Showalter SE (2010) Compassion fatigue: what is it? why does it matter? recognizing the symptoms, acknowledging the impact, developing the tools to prevent compassion fatigue and strengthen the professional already suffering from the effects. American Journal of Hospice and Palliative Medicine, 27(4), 239–242.

Singer T, Bolz M (eds.) (2013) Compassion: bridging practice and science. Munich, Germany: Max Planck Society.

Slocum-Gori S, Hemsworth D, Chan WW, Carson A, Kazajian A (2013) Understanding compassion satisfaction, compassion fatigue and burnout: a survey of the hospice palliative care workforce. Palliative Medicine, 27(2), 172–178.

Zambrano SC, Chur-Hasen A, Crawford GB (2013) The experience, coping mechanisms and impact of death and dying on palliative medicine specialists. Palliative and Supportive Care, 11, 1–8.

For further reading on the compassionate practitioner of palliative and end-of-life care, see Cassell E (2004) The nature of suffering and the goals of medicine (2nd ed.). Oxford: Oxford University Press.

To explore how compassion is demonstrated and interpreted in practice, see T Singer and M Bolz (eds.) (2013) Compassion: bridging practice and science. Munich: Max Planck Society. To understand how compassion can be fostered and sustained for the next generation of practitioners, see I Byock (2012) The best care possible: a physician's quest to transform care through the end of life. New York: Avery.

References, Bibliography, and Resources

Agosta L (2014) A rumor of empathy: reconstructing Heidegger's contribution to empathy and empathic clinical practice. Medicine, Health Care and Philosophy, 17(2): 281–292.

Antonovsky A (1979) Health, stress and coping. San Francisco: Jossey-Bass.

Aquinas T (1981) Summa theologica (transl. by the Fathers of the English Dominican Province). Westminster: Christian Classics.

Armstrong K (2009) Let's revive the Golden Rule. TED Global, July. http://www.ted.com/talks/karen_armstrong_let_s_revive_the_golden_rule

Armstrong K (2011) Twelve steps to a compassionate life. New York: Anchor.

Augé M (1995) Non-places: introduction to an anthropology of supermodernity (transl. J Howe). London: Verso.

Aulino F, Foley K (2001) The Project on Death in America. Journal of the Royal Society of Medicine, 94, 492–495.

Back AL, Bauer-Wu SM, Rushton C, Halifax J (2009) Compassionate silence in the patient-clinician encounter: a contemplative approach. Journal of Palliative Medicine, 12(12), 1113–1117.

Banks C (1990) Delicious laughter: rambunctious teaching stories from the Mathnawi Jelaluddin Rumi. Athens, GA: Maypop.

Barad J (2007) The understanding and experience of compassion: Aquinas and the Dalai Lama. Buddhist-Christian Studies, 27, 11–29.

Bergum V (2003) Relational Pedagogy. Embodiment, Improvisation and Interdependence. Nursing Philosophy, 4(2), 121–128.

Bergum V (2004) Relational ethics in nursing. In J Storch et al. (eds), Toward a moral horizon: nursing ethics for leadership and practice. Toronto, ON: Prentice Hall. 485–503.

Bern-Klug M (2004) The ambiguous dying syndrome. Health and Social Work, 29(1), 35–65.

Bethge E (1997) Dietrich Bonhoeffer: letters and papers from prison. New York: Touchstone.

Bornemark J (2014) The genesis of empathy in human development: A phenomenological reconstruction. Medicine, Health Care and Philosophy, 17(2), 259–268.

Boston PH, Mount BM (2006) The caregiver's perspective on existential and spiritual distress in palliative care. Journal of Pain and Symptom Management, 32(1), 13–26.

Boudreau JD, Cassell EJ, Fuks A (2007) A healing curriculum. Medical Education, 41, 1193–1201.

Bradshaw A (2009) Measuring nursing care and compassion: The McDonalised Nurse. Journal of Medical Ethics, 35(8), 465–468.

Bradshaw A (1996) The spiritual dimension of hospice: the secularization of an ideal. Social Science & Medicine, 43, 409–419.

Breitbart W (2008) Thoughts on the goals of psychosocial palliative care. Palliative and Supportive Care, **6**, 211–212.

Broyard A (1992) The patient examines the doctor. In Intoxicated by my illness and other writings on life and death. New York: Ballantine.

Byock I (1997) Dying well: the prospect for growth at the end of life. New York: Riverhead

Byock I (2004) The four things that matter most. 10th Anniversary Edition: A book about living. New York, Atria Books..

Byock I (2012) The best care possible: a physician's quest to transform care through the end of life. New York: Avery.

Cameron RA, Mazer BL, DeLuca JM, Mohile SG, Epstein RM (2013) In search of compassion: a new taxonomy of compassionate physician behaviours. Health Expectations. doi: 10.1111/hex.12160

Caraceni A, Grassi L (2011) Delirium: Acute confusional states in palliative medicine, Oxford, Oxford University Press.

Carr B (1999) Pity and compassion as social virtues. Philosophy, **3**, 411–429.

Cancer Pain Relief (1986) Geneva WHO Press

Cancer pain relief and palliative care (1990) Geneva, WHO Press.

Cancer pain and palliative care in children (1996) Geneva, WHO Press

Cassell E (2004) The nature of suffering and the goals of medicine (2nd ed.). Oxford: Oxford University Press.

Cassell E (2009) Suffering. In D Walsh et al. (eds.) Palliative medicine. Philadelphia: Saunders Elsevier, **9**: 46–51.

Cassell E (2014) The nature of healing: the modern practice of medicine. Oxford: Oxford University Press.

Chabner BA (1997) Cancer: a personal journey. Notes from the edge . . . The diary of Peter J. Morgan, MD. Oncologist, **2**(4), 206–207.

Cherny N, Coyle N, Foley KM (1994) Suffering in the advanced cancer patient: a definition and taxonomy. Journal of Palliative Care, **10** (2), 57–70.

Chew M, Armstrong RM, Van der Weyden MB (2003) Can compassion survive the 21st century? Editorial Medical Journal of Australia, **179**, 569–570.

Chochinov H (2007) Dignity and the essence of medicine: the A, B, C, and D of dignity conserving care. British Medical Journal, 335, 184–187.

Chochinov HM, Cann BJ (2005) Interventions to enhance the spiritual aspects of dying. Journal of Palliative Medicine, 8(Suppl 1), S103–115.

Chochinov HM, Steinstra D (2012) Vulnerability and palliative care. Palliative and Supportive Care, **10**, 1–2.

Chödrön P (2001) Start where you are: a guide to compassionate living. Boston: Shambala Classics.

Clark D (2002) Cicely Saunders: founder of the hospice movement. Selected letters, 1959–1999. Oxford: Oxford University Press.

Clark D (2005) Cicely Saunders: selected writings, 1958–2004. Oxford: Oxford University Press.

Clark D (2013) Transforming the culture of dying: the work of the Project on Death in America. Oxford: Oxford University Press.

Clark D, Small N, Wright M, Winslow M, Hughes N (2005) 'A little bit of heaven for the few?' An oral history of the modern hospice movement in the United Kingdom. Lancaster: Observatory Publications.

Cobb M (2001) The dying soul: spiritual care at the end of life. Buckingham: Open University Press.

Cohen-Katz J, Wiley D, Capuano T, Baker DM, Shapito S (2004) The effects of mindfulness-based stress reduction on nurse stress and burnout: a quantitative and qualitative study. Holistic Nursing Practice, 18(6), 302–308.

Comins M (2001) Elijah and the 'still small voice': a desert reading. CCAR Journal: A Reform Jewish Quarterly, 47(2). http://www.torahtext.org

Connor SR, (2009) Hospice and palliative care: the essential guide. New York, Routledge.

Crisp R (2008) Compassion and beyond. Ethical Theory, Morality and Practice, 11, 233–246.

Currow DC, Abernethy AP, Fazekas BS (2004) Specialist palliative care needs of whole populations: a feasibility study using a novel approach. Palliative Medicine, 18, 239–247.

Dalai Lama (2005) How to expand love: widening the circle of loving relationships. New York: Atria.

Dalai Lama (2006) Kindness, clarity, insight. Ithaca, NY: Snow Lion.

Dalai Lama (2011) How to be compassionate: a handbook for creating inner peace and a happier world. London: Atria.

Dalai Lama, Stril-Rever S (2010) My spiritual journey. New York: HarperCollins.

Dass R, Bush M (1992) Compassion in action: setting out on the path of service. New York: Bell Tower.

Davidson G (2014) The hospice: development and administration. Oxford: Routledge.

Davis C, Guyer C (2013) Integrated care pathways for dying patients—myths, misunderstandings and realities in clinical practice. European Journal of Palliative Care, 20(3), 112–119.

de Pentheny O'Kelly C, Urch C, Brown EA (2011) The impact of culture and religion on truth telling at end of life. Nephrology Dialysis Transplantation, 26, 3838–3842.

Deigh J (2004) Nussbaum's account of compassion. Philosophy and Phenomenological Research, 68(2), 465–472.

Delio I (2005) Compassion: living in the spirit of St Francis. Cincinnati, OH: Franciscan Media.

Dewar B, Adamson E, Smith S, Surfleet J, King L (2014) Clarifying misconceptions about compassionate care. Journal of Advanced Nursing, 70(8), 1738–1747.

Dodds M (1991) Thomas Aquinas, human suffering and the unchanging God of love. Theological Studies, 52, 330–344.

Downing J, Leng M, Namukwaya E, Murray S, Atieno M, Grant L (2014) Lessons from four countries in sub-Saharan African in defining and developing integrated models of palliative care. BMJ Supportive and Palliative Care, 4(1), A82–83.

Duffin C (2013) Nurses could be struck off by NMC for failing to show compassion, Nursing Standard, 27(46), 2–3.

Dumont S et al. (2014) The use of palliative sedation: a comparison of attitudes of French-speaking physicians from Quebec and Switzerland. Palliative and Supportive Care, 14, 1–9.

Egnew TR (2005) The meaning of healing: transcending suffering. Annals of Family Medicine, 3(3), 255–262.

Ekman P (2003) Emotions revealed: recognizing faces and feelings to improve communication and emotional life. New York: Henry Holt.

Famoroti TO, Fernandes L, Chima SC (2013) Stigmatization of people living with HIV/ AIDS by healthcare workers at a tertiary hospital in KwaZulu-Natal, South Africa: a cross-sectional descriptive study. BMC Medical Ethics, 14, Suppl 1, S6.

Fehr B, Sprecher S, Underwood LG (eds.) (2008) The science of compassionate love: theory, research, and applications. Malden, MA: Wiley-Blackwell.

Feldman C (2005) Compassion: listening to the cries of the world. Berkeley, CA: Rodmell.

Fernando AT, Consedine NS (2013) Beyond compassion fatigue: the transactional model of physician compassion. Journal of Pain and Symptom Management. http://dx.doi. org/10.1016/j.jpainsymman.2013.09.014

Ferrell BR, Ferrell William Ed, Ferrell William Ed (1996) Pod-Suffering: Human dimensions Pain/Illness. Burlington, Jones and Bartlett Learning.

Ferrell BR, Ferrell BA (1996) Pain in the elderly: task for on pain in the elderly. Baltimore IASP Press.

Ferrell BR, Coyne, N (2008) The nature of suffering and the goals of nursing. Oxford, Open University Press.

Figley C (ed.) (1995) Compassion fatigue: coping with secondary traumatic stress disorders in those who treat the traumatized. London: Psychology Press.

Fillion L et al. (2009) Impact of a meaning-centered intervention on job satisfaction and on quality of life among palliative care nurses. Psycho-oncology, **18**, 1300–1310.

Fillion L et al. (2013) To improve services and care at the end of life: understanding the impact of workplace satisfaction and well-being of nurses. Rapport R-794, Montréal, IRSST. http://www.irsst.qc.ca/-projet-vers-l-amelioration-des-services-et-des-soins-de-fin-de-vie-mieux-comprendre-l-impact-du-milieu-de-travail-sur-la-satisfaction-et-le-bien-etre-des-0099–6050.html

Fletcher A, Payne S, Waterman D, Turner M (2014) Palliative and end-of-life care in prisons in England and Wales—approaches taken to improve inequalities. BMJ Supportive Palliative Care, **4**, A19.

Fowler FG, Fowler HG (1964) The concise Oxford dictionary of current English. Oxford: Oxford University Press.

Fox M (1999) Spirituality named compassion: uniting mystical awareness with social justice. Rochester, VT: Inner Traditions.

Fox M (2003) Illuminations of Hildegard of Bingen. Rochester, VT: Bear & Company.

Frazer ML (2006) The compassion of Zarathustra: Nietzsche on sympathy and strength. The review of politics, **68**(1), 49–78.

Freedman R (2002) Confucius: The Golden Rule. Singapore: Scholastic Press.

Gallagher A (2013) Compassion conundrums. Nursing Ethics, **20**(8), 849–850.

Gallagher P (2009) The grounding of forgiveness: Martha Nussbaum on compassion and mercy. American Journal of Economics and Sociology, **68**(1), 231–252.

Gilbert P (2010) The compassionate mind. London: Constable.

Gilbert P (2013) Compassion-focused therapy: working with arising fears and resistances. In T Singer, M Bolz (eds.) Compassion: bridging practice and science. Munich: Max Planck Society. 112–131.

Goetz JL, Keltner D, Simon-Thomas E (2010) Compassion: an evolutionary analysis and empirical review. Psychological Bulletin, **136**(3), 351–374.

Greenleaf RK (1972) The institution as servant. Cambridge, MA: Center for Applied Studies.

Griffiths B (2001) River of compassion. Springfield, IL: Templegate.

Gustin LW, Wagner L (2013) The butterfly effect of caring—clinical nursing teachers' understanding of self-compassion as a source to compassionate care. Scandinavian Journal of Caring Sciences, **27**(1), 175–183.

Gyatso, GK (2002) Universal compassion: inspiring solutions for difficult times. New York: Tharpa.

Habermas J (1987) Theory of communicative action. Vol. II: Lifeworld and system: a critique of functionalist reason (transl. T McCarthy). Cambridge: Polity Press.

Halifax J (2008) Being with dying: cultivating compassion and fearlessness in the presence of death. New York: Shambala.

Halifax J (2011) The precious necessity of compassion. Journal of Pain and Symptom Management, **11**(1), 146–152.

Halifax J (2012) A heuristic model of enactive compassion. Current Opinion in Supportive and Palliative Care, **6**(2), 228–235.

Halifax J (2014) G.R.A.C.E. for nurses: cultivating compassion in nurse/patient interactions. Journal of Nursing Education and Practice, **4**(1), 121–128.

Halpern J (2014) From idealized clinical empathy to empathic communication in medical care. Medicine, Health Care and Philosophy, **17**(2), 301–311.

Hangartner D (2013) Human suffering and the four immeasurables: a Buddhist perspective on compassion. In T Singer, M Boltz (2013) (eds.) Compassion: bridging practice and science. Munich: Max Planck Society. Chap. 8.

Hanh TN (1995) Living Buddha, living Christ. New York: Riverhead.

Hanh TN (2009) The three jewels. A Dharma talk given 12 November. http://tnhaudio. org/2009/11/18/the-three-jewels

Harrison R, Westwood M (2009) Preventing vicarious traumatization of mental health therapists: identifying protective practices. Psychotherapy: Theory, Research, Practical Training, **46**(2), 203–219.

Hayward R (2005) Historical Keywords – Empathy. Lancet, **366**(9491), 1071.

Hebblewhite A (2014) A medical student's reflection on palliative care: managing emotional connection with patients. Palliative and Supportive Care, **27**, 1–4.

Heidegger M (2010) Being and time (rev. ed. of the Stambaugh transl.). SUNY series in contemporary continental philosophy. Albany, NY: SUNY Press.

Heschel AJ (1955) God in search of man. New York: Torchbooks.

Howell JC (2009) Introducing Christianity: exploring the Bible, faith and life (1st ed.) Louisville, KY: Westminster John Knox Press.

Ikeda D (2004) Unlocking the mysteries of birth and death . . . and everything in between: a Buddhist view of life. Santa Monica, CA: Middleway.

Illhardt FJ (2001) Scope and demarcation of palliative care In H Ten Have, R Janssens (eds) Palliative care in Europe: concepts and policies. Amsterdam: IOS Press. 109–116.

Jung C.J (2014) The collected works of C.G. Jung: complete digital edition, Adler G (Ed). New York, Princeton University Press.

Karzan B (2013) Cultivating alternative paths to compassion: generosity, forgiveness and patience. In T Singer, M Bolz (eds) Compassion: bridging practice and science. Munich: Max Planck Society.137–157.

Kearney M (1992) Palliative medicine—just another specialty? Palliative Medicine, **6**(1), 39–46.

Kearney M (2000) A place of healing: working with suffering in living and dying. Oxford: Oxford University Press.

Kearney M (2007) Mortally wounded: stories of soul pain, death, and healing (2nd ed.). New Orleans, LA: Spring Journal.

Kearney M (2009) A place of healing: working with nature and soul at the end of life. New Orleans, LA: Spring Journal.

Kearney MK, Weininger RB, Vachon MLS, Mount BM, Harrison RL (2009) Self-care of physicians caring for patients at the end of life: 'being connected . . . a key to my survival'. Journal of the American Medical Association, **301**, 1155–1164.

Keaty A (2005) The Christian Virtue of Mercy: Aquinas' transformation of Aristotelian Pity. The Heythrop Journal, **46**(2), 181–198.

Kellehear A (2013) Compassionate communities: end-of-life care as everyone's responsibility. QJM: An International Journal of Medicine, **106**(12), 1071–1075.

Kissane DW (2012) The relief of existential suffering. Archives of Internal Medicine, **172**(19), 1501–1505.

Koffman J, Camps M (2008) 'No way in': including disadvantaged population and patient groups at end-of-life. In S Payne et al. (eds) Palliative care nursing: principles and evidence for practice (2nd ed.). 362–382.

Kuah-Pearce KE (2014) Understanding suffering and giving compassion: the reach of socially engaged Buddhism in China. Anthropological Medicine, **21**(1), 27–42.

Larkin P (2011) Compassion: the essence of end-of-life care. In I Renzenbrink (ed) Caregiver stress and staff support in illness, dying and bereavement. Oxford: Oxford University Press.

Leathard HL The nature of being: a Thomistic perspective related to health and healing. Spirituality and Health International, **5**(2), 107–115.

Lewis CS (1955) Surprised by joy: the shape of my early life. Orlando, FL: Harcourt.

Lewis CS (2011) Surprised by joy/the four loves. London: Houghton Mifflin Harcourt.

Lloyd-Williams M (2009) Psychosocial care in palliative care (2nd ed.). Oxford: Oxford University Press.

Malterud K, Friedriksen L, Gjerde MH (2009) When doctors experience their vulnerability as beneficial for the patients. Scandinavian Journal of Primary Health Care, **27**, 85–90.

Mandelstam M (2006). Betraying the NHS: health abandoned. London: Jessica Kingsley.

Mathiesen M, Froggatt K, Owen E, Ashton JR (2014) End-of-life conversations in care: an asset-based model for community engagement. BMJ Supportive & Palliative Care. doi 10.1136/bmjspcare-2013-000516

Masel EK, Schur S, Watzske HH (2012) Life is uncertain, death is certain: Buddhism and palliative care. Journal of Pain and Symptom Management, **44**(2), 307–312.

Melvin CS (2012) Professional compassion fatigue: what is the true cost of nurses caring for the dying? International Journal of Palliative Nursing, **18**(12), 606–611.

Mendocal MR (2002) The ornament of the world: how Muslims, Jews and Christians created a culture of tolerance in Medieval Spain. Boston: Little Brown.

Merton T (2002) Love and living (NB Stone, Br. P Hart, eds) Boston: Houghton Mifflin Harcourt.

Mipham S (2006) Ruling your world: ancient strategies for modern life. New York: Crown Publishing Group.

Mishneh Torah [English] http://www.chabad.org

Moore T (1996) The re-enchantment of everyday life. New York: HarperCollins.

Moore T (2002) No man is an island. San Diego: Mariner.

Morrison RS (2013) Models of palliative care delivery in the United States. Current Opinion in Supportive and Palliative Care, 7(2), 201–206.

Mount B (2013) Healing, quality of life and the need for a paradigm shift in palliative care. Journal of Palliative Care, 29(1), 45–48.

Mount B, Kearney M (2003) Healing and palliative care: charting our way forward. Palliative Medicine, **17**, 657–658.

Muhammad T (2014) Islam on mercy and compassion. London: Minhaj-Ul-Quran.

Myers GE (2003) Restoration or transformation? choosing ritual strategies for end-of-life care. Mortality, **8**(4), 372–387.

Myers GE Mount BM, Boston PH, Cohen SR (2007) Healing connections: on moving from suffering to a sense of well-being. Journal of Pain and Symptom Management, **33**(4), 372–388.

Neff K (2011) Self-compassion: the proven power of being kind to yourself. New York: William Morrow.

Neff K, Germer C (2013a) Being kind to yourself: the science of self-compassion in T Singer, M Bolz (eds) Compassion: bridging practice and science. Munich: Max Planck Society. 492–499.

Newdick C, Danbury C (2013) Culture, compassion and clinical neglect: Probity in the NHS after Mid Staffordshire. Journal of Medical Ethics, Published Online First, 08.04.14, doi.1010.1136/medethics.2012-101048.

Neff KD, Germer CK (2013b) A pilot study and randomized controlled trial of the mindful self-compassion program. Journal of Clinical Psychology, **69**(1), 28–44.

Nilsson P (2011) On the suffering of compassion. Philosophia, **39**, 125–144.

Nouwen H (1979) The wounded healer: Ministry in contemporary society. Colorado, Image Books

Nouwen HJM, McNeill DP, Morrison DA (1982) Compassion: a reflection on the Christian life. New York: Doubleday.

Nussbaum MC (1996) Compassion: the basic social emotion. Social Philosophy and Policy, **13**, 27–58.

Nussbaum MC (2001) Upheavals in thought: the intelligence of emotions. Cambridge: Cambridge University Press.

O'Donohue J (2003) Divine beauty: the invisible embrace. London: Bantam.

Owain Hughes T (2013) The compassion quest. London: SPCK.

Paley J (2013) Social psychology and compassion deficit. Nurse Education Today, **33**, 1451–1452.

Pask E (2003) Moral agency in Nursing" Seeing value in the work and believing that I make a difference. Nursing Ethics, **10**(2), 165–174.

Peabody FW (1927) The care of the patient. Journal of the American Medical Association, **88**, 876–882.

Penman J, Oliver M, Harrington A (2013) The relational model of spiritual engagement depicted by palliative care clients and caregivers. International Journal of Nursing Practice, **19**(1), 39–46.

Penrod J, Loed SJ, Smith CA (2009) Administrators' perspectives on changing practice in end-of-life care in a state prison system. Public Health Nursing, **31**(2), 99–108.

Perget P, Lützén K (2012) Balancing truth-telling in the preservation of hope: a relational ethics approach. Nursing Ethics, **19**(1), 21–29.

Peteet JR, Balboni MJ (2013) Spirituality and religion in oncology. CA: A Cancer Journal for Clinicians, **63**, 280–289.

Picardie R, Seaton M, Picardie J (1997) Before I say goodbye: recollections and observations for one woman's final year. New York: Henry Holt & Company.

Pollock A (2004). NHS plc: the privatisation of our health care. Bath: Verso.

Post SG, Underwood LG, Schloss JP, Hurlbut WB (eds.) (2002) Altruism and altruistic love: science, philosophy, and religion in dialogue. New York: Oxford University Press.

Quill TE, Cassel CK (1995) Nonabandonment: a central obligation for physicians. Annals of Journal of Medicine, **122**(5), 368–374.

Rabow MW, Carrie NE, Remen RN (2013) Repression of personal values and qualities in medical education. Family Medicine, **45**(1), 13–18.

Radbruch L, deLima L, Lohmann D, Gwyther E, Payne S (2013) The Prague Charter: urging governments to relieve suffering and ensure the right to palliative care. Palliative Medicine, **27**(2), 101–102.

Randall F, Downie RS (2006) The philosophy of palliative care: critique and reconstruction. Oxford: Oxford University Press.

Reeves NC (2011) Death acceptance through ritual. Death Studies, **35**, 408–419.

Registered Nurses' Association of Ontario (2013). Developing and sustaining interprofessional health care: optimizing patients/clients, organizational, and system outcomes. Toronto, ON: Registered Nurses' Association of Ontario.

Remen RN (2001) My grandfather's blessings: stories of strength, refuge and belonging. New York: Riverhead.

Remen RN (2006) Kitchen table wisdom. New York: Riverhead.

Remen RN (2008) Practicing a medicine of the whole person: an opportunity for healing. Hematology/Oncology Clinics of North America, **22**(4), 767–773.

Renzenbrink I (ed.) (2011) Caregiver stress and staff support in illness, dying and bereavement. Oxford: Oxford University Press.

Rich BA (2014) Prognosis terminal: truth-telling in the context of end-of-life care. Cambridge Quarterly of Healthcare Ethics, **23**, 209–219.

Riess H, Kelley JM, Bailey RW, Dunn EJ, Phillips M (2012) Empathy training for resident physicians: a randomized controlled trial of a neuroscience-informed curriculum. Journal of General Internal Medicine, **27**(10), 1280–1286. doi 10.1007/s 11606-012-2063.2

Rinpoche S, Gaffney P, Harvey A (2012) The Tibetan book of living & dying: the spiritual classic and international bestseller. San Francisco: Harper.

Rinpoche CN, Shima D (2006) Medicine and compassion: a Tibetan lama's guidance for caregivers. Somerville, MA: Wisdom Publications.

Rivett G (1998) From cradle to grave: 50 years of the NHS. London: King's Fund.

Rogers C (1951) Client-centered therapy: its current practice, implications and theory. London: Constable.

Rogers CR, Stevens B, Gendlin ET, Shlien JM, Van Dusen W (1967) Person to person: the problem of being human: a new trend in psychology. Lafayette, CA: Real People Press.

Running A, Woodward Tolle L, Girard D (2008) Ritual: the final expression of care. International Journal of Nursing Practice, **14**, 303–307.

Sabo B (2008) Adverse psychological consequences: compassion fatigue, burnout and vicarious traumatization: are nurses who provide palliative and haematological cancer care vulnerable? Indian Journal of Palliative Care, **14**, 23–29.

Sanchez-Reilly S, Morrison LJ, Casey E, Bernacki R, O'Neill L, Kopo J (2013) Caring for oneself to care for others: physicians and their self-care. Journal of Supportive Oncology, **11**(2), 75–81.

Saslow LR et al. (2013) The social significance of spirituality: new perspectives on the compassion-altruism relationship. Psychology of Religion and Spirituality, **5**(3), 201–218.

Sasser CG, Pulchalski CM (2010) The humanistic clinician: traversing the science and art of health care. Journal of Pain and Symptom Management, **39**(5), 936–940.

Saunders C (1996) Into the valley of the shadow of death: a personal therapeutic journey. British Medical Journal, **7072**(313), 1599–1601.

Saunders C (2003) Watch with me: inspiration for a life in hospice care. London: Mortal Press.

Saunders C (2005) Foreword. In J Ling, L O'Sioráin (eds.) Palliative care in Ireland. Facing Death Series. Berkshire: Open University Press. xix–xxii.

Schantz M (2007) Compassion: a concept analysis. Nursing Forum **42**(2), 48–55.

Schildman E, Schildman J (2014) Palliative sedation therapy: a systematic literature review and critical appraisal of available guidance on motivation and decision-making. Journal of Palliative Medicine, **17**(5), 601–611.

Sears D (1998) Compassion for humanity in the Jewish tradition. Northvale, NJ: Jason Aronson.

Seeds of Compassion (2008) The Desmond Tutu Peace Foundation. http://www.tutufoundation-usa.org

Seno VL (2010) Being-with dying: authenticity in end-of-life encounters. American Journal of Hospice and Palliative Medicine, **27**(6), 377–386.

Sevensky RL (1983) The religious foundations of health care: a conceptual approach. Journal of Medical Ethics, **9**, 165–169.

Shanafelt, TD, West C, Zhao X, Novotny P, Kolars J, Habernmann T, Sloan J (2005) Relationship between increased personal well-being and enhanced empathy among internal medicine residents. Journal of General Internal Medicine, **20**(7), 559–564.

Shapiro SL, Astin JA, Bishop SR, Cordova M (2005) Mindfulness-based stress reduction for health care professionals: results from a randomized trial. International Journal of Stress Management, **12**(2), 164–176.

Showalter SE (2010) Compassion fatigue: what is it? why does it matter? recognizing the symptoms, acknowledging the impact, developing the tools to prevent compassion fatigue and strengthen the professional already suffering from the effects. American Journal of Hospice and Palliative Medicine, **27**(4), 239–242.

Singer T, Bolz M (eds.) (2013) Compassion: bridging practice and science. Munich, Germany: Max Planck Society.

Smajdor A (2013) Should compassionate care be incentivised? Nursing Times, **109**, 49–50.

Slocum-Gori S, Hemsworth D, Chan WW, Carson A, Kazajian A (2013) Understanding compassion satisfaction, compassion fatigue and burnout: a survey of the hospice palliative care workforce. Palliative Medicine, **27**(2), 172–178.

Soyannwo O (2014) Pain management in sub-Saharan Africa: innovative approaches to improving access. Pain Management, **4**(1), 5–7.

Sprecher S, Fehr B (2005) Compassionate love for close others and humanity. Journal of Social and Personal Relationships, **22**, 629–651.

St Teresa of Avila (2010) The interior castle (study ed.; transl. K Kavanaugh, O Rodriguez). Washington: ICS.

Stanworth R, Saunders CD (2004) Recognizing spiritual needs in people who are dying. Oxford: Oxford University Press.

Steinhauser KE, Christakis NA, Clipp EC, McNeilly M, McINtyre L, Tulsky JA (2000) Factors considered important at the end-of-life by patients, family, physicians and other care providers. Journal of the American Medical Association, **284**(19), 2476–2482.

Stienstra D, Chochinov HM (2007) Palliative care for vulnerable populations. Palliative and Supportive Care, **10**, 37–42.

Storr A (2013) The essential Jung: selected and introduced by Anthony Storr (reissue ed.). New York: Princeton University Press.

Svenaeus F (2014) The phenomenology of empathy in medicine: an introduction. Medicine, Health Care and Philosophy, **17**, 245–248.

Swinton J (2007) Raging with compassion: pastoral responses to the problem of evil. Cambridge: William B. Eerdmans.

Ten Boom C, Sherill J, Sherill E (1984) The hiding place. London: Bantam.

Teno J, Connor S (2011) Referring a patient and family to high-quality palliative care at the close of life: 'We met a new personality . . . with this level of compassion and empathy.' In S McPhee et al. (eds.) Care at the close of life: evidence and experience. New York: McGraw Hill. 523–536.

The practice of loving-kindness (Mettā): as taught by the Buddha in the Pali Canon (comp. and transl. Ñ Thera) (2013) Access to insight (legacy ed.), 30 November http://www.accesstoinsight.org/lib/authors/nanamoli/wheel007.html

Thomas of Celano (2000) The first life of St Francis of Assisi. New York: Triangle.

Tutu D, Allen J (2010) God is not a Christian: speaking truth in times of crisis. London: Rider.

Tutu D, Tutu M (2014) The book of forgiving: the fourfold path for healing ourselves and our world. New York: HarperCollins.

Vachon MLS (1978) Motivation and stress experienced by staff working with the terminally ill. Reprinted in GW Davidson (ed.) The hospice: development and administration. Washington: Hemisphere.

Vachon MLS (1995) Staff stress in hospice/palliative care: a review. Palliative Medicine, **9**(2), 91–122.

Vachon MLS (2009) The emotional problems of the patient in palliative medicine. In G Hanks et al. (eds) Oxford textbook of palliative medicine (4th ed.). Oxford: Oxford University Press. 1410–1436.

Vachon MLS (2011) Four decades of selected research in hospice/palliative care: have the stressors changed? In I Renzenbrink (ed.) Caregiver stress and staff support in illness, dying, and bereavement. Oxford: Oxford University Press. 1–24.

Vachon MLS (2012) Reflections on compassion, suffering and occupational stress. In J Malpas, N Lickiss (eds) Perspectives on human suffering. Dordrecht, The Netherlands: Springer. 317–331.

Wallerstedt B, Benzein E, Andershead B (2011) Sharing living and dying: a balancing act between vulnerability and a sense of security: enrolled nurses' experience of working in the sitting service for dying patients at home. Palliative and Supportive Care, **9**, 295–303.

Walsh D, Foley KM, Caraceni A, Fainsinger R, Glare P, Goh C, Lloyd-Williams M, Nunez-Olarte J, Radbruch L (2008) Palliative Medicine, Expert Consult. Philadelphia, WB Saunders Company.

Weissman D (2011) Martyrs in palliative care. Journal of Palliative Medicine, **14**(12), 1278–1279.

Weng H, Fox AS, Shackman AJ, Stodola DE, Caldwell JZK, Rogers GM, Davidson RJ (2013) Compassion training alters altruism and neural responses to suffering. Psychological Science, **24**(7), 1171–1180.

Whitebrook M (2002) Compassion as a political virtue. Political Studies, **50**(3), 529–544.

Wigglesworth C (2012) SQ21: the twenty-one skills of spiritual intelligence. New York, Selectbooks

Wilson F, Ingleton C, Gott M, Gardner C (2014) How do perceptions of risk shape 'choice' in end-of-life care. BMJ Supportive Palliative Care, **4**, Suppl 1, A 28.

Winnicott DW (1953) Transitional objects and transitional phenomenon—a study of first not-me possession. International Journal of Psycho-Analysis, **34**, 89–97.

Wishart PM (2005) Conceptualising compassionate power. Spirituality and Health International, **6**(1), 33–38.

Wolterstorff N (2002) Lament for a son. The Living Pulpit, October-December, 13.

World Health Organisation (2002) Palliative care. http://www.who.int/cancer/palliative/definition/en/

Wright B (2004) Compassion fatigue: how to avoid it [editorial]. Palliative Medicine, **18**, 3–4.

Wright R (2010) The evolution of God. Boston: Back Bay Books.

Youngson R (2008) Compassion in health care: the missing dimension of healthcare reform. The NHS Confederation Futures Debate, paper 2. www.debatepapers.org.uk

Youngson R (2012) Time to care: how to love your patients and your job. Raglan, NZ: Rebelheart.

Zambrano SC, Chur-Hasen A, Crawford GB (2013) The experience, coping mechanisms and impact of death and dying on palliative medicine specialists. Palliative and Supportive Care, **11**, 1–8.

Zimmerman C (2012) Acceptance of dying: a discourse analysis of palliative care literature. Social Science & Medicine, **75**(1), 217–224.

Additional web resources

The e-book *Compassion: Bridging Practice and Science*, edited by Tania Singer and Matthias Bolz (2013) can be downloaded free from. http://www.compassion-training.org. The book provides a comprehensive interactive resource about the art and science of compassion. It can be downloaded to PC or Mac but is designed for best use on iPads.

Some of the authors cited in this book have web pages which highlight other publications and resources which may be of interest:

◆ Sharon Salzberg: http://www.sharonsalzberg.com

◆ Rachel Naomi Remen: http://wwwrachelremen.com

◆ Caroline Myss: http://www.myss.com

Information on the work of Commonweal can be accessed at http://www.rachelremen.com.

The footprints poem cited in the chapter on Mary Vachon can be downloaded at: http://footprints.in.the.sand.com

The Registered Nurses' Association of Ontario's inter-professional practice guidelines are available at http://www.rnao.ca/bpg/guidelines/interprofessional-team-work-healthcare

Index

DATE DUE

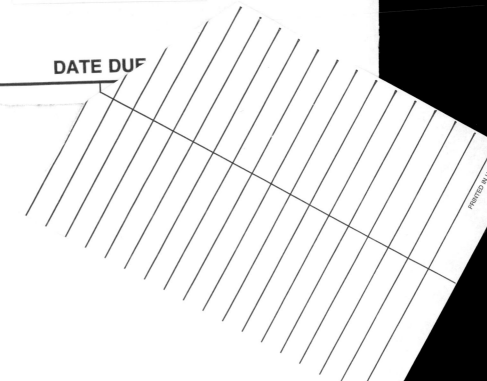

PRINTED IN U.S.A.